A CANCEROUS TRANSFORMATION

EVAN ORTLIEB, PH.D.

A Cancerous Transformation

Evan Ortlieb, Ph.D.

'Competitive by nature, loving by necessity, and dedicated by choice'

This book is dedicated to everyone who has been affected by cancerous diseases.

Cuthroat   Cancer is a relentless disease. Without the combination of excellent oncologists, loving friends and family, healthcare, and God, the outcome is bleak.

Asinine   The thought of someone choosing to live a lifestyle that promotes and spreads carcinogenic substances to the body.

Nausea   Feeling nauseous is an inevitable and unrelenting consequence of stepping up to the plate and choosing chemotherapy treatment to wage a battle with a cancerous disease within the body.

Caveat   Cancer often shows its face when one least expects it, so it is always critical for one to live to the fullest in the meantime.

Energizing   Kinship provides cancer patients with the desire and spirit to continue their fight for life, so show that you care every chance you get.

Refusal   The only way to conquer cancer is through utter determination; never accept its power over one's own. Those who have won the battle with cancer are cancer 'defeators', not cancer survivors.

Table of Contents

Prelude

If you have chosen to begin reading this book, it is likely that cancer has shown its ugly face to someone you know, if not yourself. This text began as a compilation of my life struggles and conquests, but developed into much more. Its content is shared exactly how I remember, serving as a collection of experiences from the lives of many individuals. My life has taken strides from one point in time to the next, sometimes connected and at others without any transition periods at all.

This book was not written to brighten one's perspective or leave the reader feeling better upon its conclusion, but instead directed at challenging human emotion and feeling. My aims include trying to address issues that include 'what does chemotherapy feel like?' and 'how can one care for others who are undergoing chemotherapy?' It is also my hope that from this manuscript, readers will reflect upon their own lives. I am but 30 something years old, yet I have seen, felt, and witnessed a life full of pleasure and pain.

When contemplating a beginning point for this text, I realized that I had to address my background, as it provides the structure that shapes who I am. Being raised in a middle-class Catholic family, I had all the necessities of life—good schooling, loving parents, and a tight-knit family as well as a host of friends. Life was ordinary by all means . . .

Chapter 1:

Everyday Life

Every stage of life has its perks and hardships; the teenage years are like no other—full of opportunities to excel in any aspect of life including fine arts, drama, music, sports, and academics. All of these can fully manifest without having most of the responsibilities that come with adulthood. Generally people fall into two categories: those who love their adolescence and those who wish to forget it. For me, it was as simple as—go to school, work for spending money, and have as much enjoyment as possible. Every day was an opportunity to develop skills and interests that would have laid the groundwork for my future, if only I had utilized my efforts appropriately. In fact, being a teenager was relatively easy . . . in hindsight.

Try telling that to a 16-year-old boy though. No teenager who has a thousand ideas encircling his mind would concur. Impressing the guys and gaining popularity with the girls are major concerns. My hair is growing too long and needs to be cut. My jeans are getting worn to the point where there are holes in them, even though that is a trendy style to some. My shirts aren't a popular name brand unless you count Wal-Mart as a designer name. Status and support from others are the most sought after goals by many high school students—an unfortunate state of affairs. Whether it comes from appearance, dress, or popularity, teenagers have their hands full when it comes to trying to manage a host of complexities, which are much easier to analyze now as an outsider. Still, decisions and actions are made in the present and thus, they are not always rational but instead a result of emotions. Hormonal fluxes, peer pressure, and self-establishment of individual personalities provide ample reason why these years are exceptionally difficult to navigate. The decisions that teenagers make though often have longstanding effects on their way of life by establishing norms, tendencies, habits, beliefs, and comfort levels. And the results . . . well the results are not always advantageous—to which anyone who has surpassed those years can readily attest.

School

My life has always revolved around school, and it always will. But before I get to that, you will need to understand my experiences as a 16 year old. About what did I worry, spend my time doing, and consider dear to my heart? As you will see, all of these answers were clearly centered on me. Others' concerns were just that—for others with which to deal. My concerns, though, were for everyone to manage. This narrow-minded perspective was one that I regret today, but it was in full-force during my adolescence.

(6:00 a.m.) BUZZ! BUZZ! Ahhhhh, I am so tired, "Just five more minutes." Please let me hit the snooze button a couple of times. Sometimes I asked my father, Robert, for more time to sleep; other times I begged God to make it be the weekend so I could sleep in until any random time in the afternoon. Getting ready for high school in the morning was a pain to say the least. Why couldn't school hours be from 12:00PM to 3:00PM? Regular folks could actually make it to school on time, remain well-rested, and still put in a few hours of studious work per day. Eating cereal, putting on some clothes, and hopping in the car for my father to drive me to school does not sound like a rigorous protocol; still, it felt grueling. I suppose staying up until late hours of the night did not bode well for feeling energetic the next day. This was the daily grind that I lived and as you can distinguish, life was overbearingly difficult to my sheltered mind.

My cash flow, or lack thereof, was another common obstacle. Securing monies on a regular basis involved performing yard work for residents in the neighborhood in which I lived. Yet, this source of income was more seasonal than I preferred. Winter time came and my income died like the fallen leaves during those months. As a result, it was necessary to obtain a position as a regular employee of a company in the area. Without owning a vehicle it was essential that the job would be within walking distance, so naturally the nearest fast food restaurant chain was an obvious option. The company was known in the area for hiring young high school students. I had inside knowledge of this information because my brother, Erich, who is almost two years older than me, had already obtained a job there one year prior to my inquiry. I found myself going through a painstaking interview process that consisted of the following conversation:

Manager: So you are interested in working here?

Evan: Yes

Manager: When can you start?

Evan: As soon as possible

I was ready to enter into the real-world of Corporate America. My boss at this establishment set my schedule each week so that I would work from 7:00AM-5:00PM on Saturdays. Even before I began working, it was apparent that my work hours and school hours combined with my tendencies of being a night owl would negatively contribute to my health. Often I found myself feeling awful when awakening for work, typically only having slept for three to four hours. A 10-hour shift was a bit much for a weekend, I thought. Yet, this would allow me to earn $5.15 per hour times 10. Now that was some real money! Compared to my brother's salary who had been working there for about a year, he was only making 20 cents more per hour. What a way to reward company employees and encourage loyalty.

My weekly battles between going to work to earn some extra cash and staying in bed to recoup some vitality were epic. Sometimes, the bed won outright. This struggle to maintain the first component of transitioning into adulthood, holding down a job, was ongoing each and every week. One would think that naturally the body would adjust to waking up each Saturday at 6:15AM, but it never did. Even at work, I used every excuse to rest if even for a moment. "I'll take out the trash," was a commonly-uttered ploy to go outside for 5 to 10 minutes of relaxation. In an environment where mice ran rampant and the stench was awful, I was in solace. Emptying the trash was my favorite part of the job because it was the most tranquil. My body was like an engine not firing on all cylinders, which did not mesh well in the fast-paced environment of yelling, "Where are the fries?" and "You need to drop some baskets." Buzzers sounded every 20 seconds when the meat patties were ready to be scraped off the grill, while others rang when pieces of fried chicken were to be collected from grease vats that regularly burned and scarred my hands. Meanwhile, upper management had the gall to yell at me about shortages of hash browns or French Fries. I was not in the mood nor had the tolerance for all this mayhem at 7:00AM on Saturdays. I kept thinking about telling one or all of the bosses, "I'll trade positions with you any day . . . just let me know." But I kept my thoughts inside and refrained from voicing my sentiments.

School and work were center figures in my life much like any other adolescent. While some students attend high school to study, learn, and make friendships that last a lifetime, I saw high school as a place to act foolishly to impress classmates. Shenanigans was my middle name. Cracking jokes aimed at fellow students and

14

being mischievous were my chosen methods of gaining popularity. Sometimes, it involved critiquing students based on their appearances. "Hey Cereal Box!" was one example of my persecution of another student who had an irregularly shaped head. Other instances incorporated talking about how vastly inferior others' athletic abilities were when compared to my perceived superiority in a range of sports from basketball to golf. Again, I am not proud of some of my actions throughout various stages of life, but telling the absolute truth is necessary for you to see through my eyes.

One of the hundreds of practical jokes committed was directed towards my high school's administration. It involved creating a unique parking tag for my older brother's newly acquired vehicle during his senior year of high school. I had rights to use it on occasion, but it was basically his to drive. Parking spaces were a premium at school and only issued at the first of the school year. Therefore, it seemed logical to just make our own. Rumor had it that the parking tags were not even checked that closely, so it seemed like a no-brainer. I folded several sheets of paper, taped the edges down, cut the proper shape, and voila—I had a parking tag. Instead of it saying, "Property of Baton Rouge Magnet High School---

Student Parking Pass," ours said, "I park where I please"—a direct and candid statement that got our point across in our opinion. Sure enough, my brother drove us to school the following day. I hung the tag on the rearview mirror and we went to class. During third period that day, an announcement was made to the entire school on the intercom system: "Would the owner of a gray, Toyota Camry, license plate number XXX-XXXX, come to the front office immediately?" I did not think anything of it and then it hit me. Oh crap! That is our car. They must have noticed the tag and became furious about our self-serving confidence and swagger. Just 45 seconds later, my brother entered my Physics classroom, stood in front of me, and began conversing about how he was a senior and would be taking the rap for the infraction. Meanwhile, Mrs. Cao was still trying to teach the class. That was the craziest part . . . the lack of concern that my brother had for her instruction. Nevertheless, he eventually went down to the office, where he was grilled by the principal about his callous behavior. Erich was issued an after-school detention, which he served later in the week. My punishment was non-existent once again.

Social interactions of all kinds were the life of high school; academic achievement was of secondary or tertiary importance. Growing up in a household where academics were stressed, I also knew the value of attaining high grades. It was just that I did not feel like exerting much effort, so I lived by the minimalist motto—do whatever I needed in order to receive grades that were good enough for my parents. I was content making a 3.5 grade point average (GPA); after all, I did not have to crack a book to study or spend countless hours doing homework like my brother. Notice how I used the phrase, "making a 3.5 GPA," and not earning a 3.5 GPA. Spending my free time watching television, roaming the neighborhood, or playing poor-man's golf in a field down the road were much more exciting than reading, writing, and engaging in school-based activities.

Class time was sometimes spent completing homework at the last second before it was due. Since I never wrote down my homework assignments, I relied on my memory. This systematic method was neither effective nor functional. I rarely did any work at home so when class time came, I was in serious trouble . . . at least theoretically. Being a quick-witted lad, I always came up with what I thought were ingenious methods to get around the rules presented to me. For instance, in 11th grade English class, there were countless texts, stories, and other pieces of literature that were assigned as homework. Reading responses were one of the primary methods by which the teacher evaluated whether or not students read the material and to what extent the information was understood. On one day in particular, I entered the classroom hearing the teacher state, "Get out your homework . . . I am coming around to check it." Those are words that generally bring panic to non-compliant students, but not me. I went into action. Instead of sitting where I normally did, I shifted seats to sit on the opposite side of the classroom. There, I hurriedly jotted down some nonsensical answers that would merely represent writing on the page to complete the homework before the teacher got to that side of the room. Having to hide the fact that I was writing down answers was also a factor that elevated the difficulty of this undertaking. Sure enough, the teacher arrived at my desk and after glancing over my written answers, I received a check for the day. Yes! Hooray, for my efforts were worthwhile and led to my further conditioning that this dishonest practice was perfectly acceptable. By all accounts, I perceived it to be mission

18

accomplished. Collecting these necessary homework points, which I considered to be gimme points, boosted my grades from not performing well on the tests, which were based on that same material with which I did not read. As a result, I went back into my toolkit, looking for alternative techniques to attain greater success on the examinations.

On another memorable occasion, being a sometimes absent-minded individual, I was clueless about an apparent physics project that was due. The realization only occurred upon my arrival to class the day it was due. Missing 40 points on an incomplete project seemed like an abnormally large penalty for simply forgetting about an assignment. I was not prepared to swallow that outcome. What was I to do? Having an elderly substitute teacher that day gave me some time and opportunity to conjure a scheme. The best plan I determined was to borrow someone else's project, take it to the copy machine, and photocopy the project in its entirety, white out the name, and turn it in as my own. Besides, she probably will not even read these projects in depth. It seemed to be foolproof, that is, when using my over-confident and sometimes cocky mindset.

How it played out was quite contrary to how I envisioned receiving full credit for the assignment. In all, there were two fools: the classmate who allowed me to copy his paper, and me, the one who copied the work. Both of us received zero credit on this 40-point assignment. I thought the punishment was a bit harsh for both parties. Had I known about the assignment, I would have completed it without reservation. For whatever reason, from that time forward the physics teacher seemed to hold a grudge against me, taking additional points from my grade on group assignments in which my partners and I did the same work, leading to my only C in high school. I wonder why?

Not every instance of mischief ended with negative results, thank goodness. One particular day, in an instant, I learned a lifelong lesson about cheating in school and as a result, my habit was curbed. My drive and desire to succeed became central focus, as opposed to getting by with minimal or no work at all. Thank you, Mrs. Gregoire. I appreciate that lesson for which I am entirely grateful for learning. It has changed my life forever.

During a test in English III, I could not understand or interpret the meaning of a question. I rose from my seat and began walking to the teacher's desk to inquire and hopefully receive clarification. As I approached Mrs. Gregoire's desk, a small piece of paper began to fall from my lap. Glancing down as the small slip of paper fluttered like at a ticker-tape parade, time stood still. It finally floated down landing beside my feet. My heart was beating so hard it could likely be seen from outside my shirt! Thinking, "Oh my God, you idiot!" I swallowed, looked up, and met eyes with the teacher. She looked down and immediately arose from her desk. Mrs. Gregoire walked in front of me, picked up the piece of paper, and said, "Evan, is this yours?" With my eyes bugging out of my head and my heart pounding away, I said, "Huh, no." Then, she asked what it was that I wanted in approaching her desk. To only exacerbate the problematic situation, I had forgotten what I was going to ask her by that time. In a terrified craze, I made up a question that seemed at best half-way relevant. She gave me a simplistic answer, telling me to return to my desk. While narrowly avoiding soiling my pants, I thought, "Great . . . I am in deep shit right about now. She surely busted me." Trying not to look up, I continued navigating the remainder of the test while perspiring profusely. Without being noticed, I glanced upward to see what Mrs.

Gregoire was doing back at her desk with the piece of paper, also known as my cheat sheet. This slip of paper had all kinds of information about the characters in the book that were typed and printed using a font size 4—a technique I had mastered over the years in English I, French I and II, and even various math classes. I timidly watched as the teacher read its contents. The action that followed blew me away completely. She dropped the slip of paper in the trash receptacle.

This incident was never brought up by the teacher or ever mentioned again. Interestingly enough, the following day, two students took make-up tests in that same English class. Those two students were caught cheating in the hallway and in return, they received zeros on their tests. Somehow, I managed to receive an A on the test, even though I did not deserve it. From that instant in Mrs. Gregoire's class, I vowed to never take inappropriate routes toward desired goals. With my attitudinal change towards academics intact, achievements followed soon thereafter.

After-school

Once the bell rang to indicate the end of the school day, or even before at times, I felt free to leave school to do what I really wanted like play computer games and go golfing with my friends. Many times, the same high jinks that I pursued in school continued afterwards. Mostly our antics revolved around the golf course for a variety of reasons: 1) We loved playing golf, 2) It provided an opportunity to bamboozle many people back to back while circling the fringe of the course in a vehicle, and 3) Two golf courses were located within 2 miles of our high school—that good ole Baton Rouge Magnet High for which we proudly proclaimed.

Drive-bys. In the golfing community, drive-bys are a golfer's worst nightmare and an immature teenagers' best friend. They consist of a passerby making disruptive noises as a golfer is teeing off or swinging to hit a shot during the course of play. Every golfer has received his fair share of these instances, notwithstanding those who only play at posh country clubs. Whether it was honking a horn just prior to a golfer making contact with the ball or yelling "MISS IT" as loud as we could, drive-bys were classic examples of the simple, sadistic pleasures we as teenagers took in screwing with others.

My rambunctious friends and I participated in many acts of injustice beyond those trivial matters already mentioned. Tim, Ira,

Erich, and I were inseparable. The following is another snippet of our mischief. Golf carts were viewed as the epitome of luxury for high school students without any money. We played on courses with the cheapest greens fees in the city, which we couldn't readily afford and thus never paid them. On top of that, we spited those who could afford to rent golf carts for their round of golf while we walked the course each and every time we played. When the opportunity arose, we took full advantage of using a golf cart in an inappropriate manner. We decided to take one of the golf carts for a leisure ride all over the course with four boys sitting, standing, and hanging off every side. How did we do this? Someone from our group mysteriously found a key to a golf cart in the clubhouse behind the counter on the key rack. It came as quite a surprise that a key was found there. Of course, no harm was meant by any of our actions; the intent was just to be rebellious. Still, some people were obviously offended by our actions, as a man chased us from the clubhouse running full-speed after us. Once we discovered someone was the wiser, I stomped the gas pedal. Only seconds later we realized that the electric cart had not been fully charged and was about to run out of power. We ran in all different directions as we

24

ditched the vehicle; meanwhile, the clubhouse worker yelled at us saying that we would be arrested. Eventually, each of us snuck back to our vehicle and drove away. Even though we met these instances of confrontation, they did not stop us from continuing to be roguish. It became so habitual that I was eventually banned from the golf course on two separate occasions—a record for which I was pleased to hold.

But before the bannings, we wanted to raise the ante. Like any other type of behavior, doing the same things over and over became less fulfilling over time. Our tolerance for absurd behavior was becoming quite high. Staying on the golfing theme, we sometimes frequented the local putt-putt facility. We drove there, over-packing a friend's car full of male adolescents. Arriving at our destination with little to no money never prevented us from playing. With our big smiles intact, we knew that we would not only have a tremendous time but also leave with more than which we came. The number of putt-putt golf balls that we borrowed ranged from 1 to 73 per visitation. These outings led us to conjecture about how we could use these golf balls in some productive manner.

Several days later, while riding in Tim's car again, we thought it would be amusing to drive by the golf course. We determined that the perfect utility of the putt-putt balls would be to exchange them for golfers' balls in mid-play. Our vehicle approached various holes on the golf course before we saw our victim. On a whim I jumped out of the slowly moving vehicle while beside the 10th hole at a favorite course of ours. A man had just hit from the fairway and his golf ball landed on the green about 100 yards in front of where he currently stood. I darted out in front of the man and proceeded to run down the middle of the fairway toward the green. Of course, the man had no idea what I was doing at the time, but by the time he reached the green, his ball was now a pink, putt-putt golf ball instead of his white Titleist. Mission accomplished! We had just swindled this guy and he did not even see it coming. Running off the green towards a side-street where my friend's car was approaching provided me a quick getaway. We cruised off victoriously right down the dead-end road.

"Yeahhhhh, sucker!" Laughing and high-fiving all around, we quickly realized that we were headed for disaster—right to a dead end. "Oh crap! Let's see if we can back up, turn around, and head outta here before the guy even notices." So as we began back towards the direction we came, up and over a ridge in the road, we saw something rather startling. The golfer whose ball we stole was standing in the middle of the road with his golf club raised, as if he were in a movie like *Gangs of New York*. It was obvious to all that the man was exceedingly perturbed at our actions, as he stood pounding the club into the palm of his hand. His mannerisms clearly indicated to us that a confrontation was almost a certainty. Of the four individuals in the car, Tim, Ira, Erich, and me, there was plenty of unutilized intelligence to go around. My proposed idea was that I could hang out of the trunk while blocking the license plate with my hands so the man could not write down the tag information. Someone else said we should cover it with a towel, but I knew the wind would just blow it up. Then, Tim realized that he had a handy screwdriver with which we immediately used to remove the license plate from the vehicle. Of course, we realized that it was illegal to drive without the vehicle's tag identification, but the alternative of getting identified seemed far more likely of having detrimental outcomes. Once the plate was removed, we drove up to the ridge and down the road. By this time, the man was standing beside the street with a pen and paper, just as we had suspected. As intelligent-minded as he was, the four bandits were yet again one step ahead in the game. We drove by at a regular rate of speed. As we passed the man who was prepared to jot down the license plate number, we turned our heads to see the look on the man's face; it was priceless. His face changed from 'Now, I've got these kids' to 'Son of a bitch.' Meanwhile, Ira yelled out the car window, "Screw you old man!" Wow. It was a spectacle to behold. Driving away from the scene was a joyous occasion. Only a block down the road, we pulled into the nearest condominium complex, refastened the license plate, and drove off into the sunset. We had another story to boost our reputation of adolescent naughtiness when conversing with our friends at school. This event was etched into our memories forever.

Ironically, I was captain of the golf team as a junior in high school that same year. So at the same time that we were terrorizing golfers, I was playing in high school golf tournaments. Only a crazy-minded individual would act in this manner while supposedly serving as a role model to his teammates. My school's team, much like other high school teams in Baton Rouge, was comprised of a mixture of talent. I proudly won almost every one of the tournaments held at the same golf course from which I was banned, which was quite amusing.

Although I was a decent golfer, I began to feel the pressure to continue winning tournaments from my loved ones. I had about a two handicap in golfing terms at the age of 16. Although I practiced regularly, I knew that I had many areas in which to improve. Family and friends expected me to win and on those few occasions when I did not, I heard about it.

Joey: "How much did you win by today?"

Evan: "Actually, I got second place."

Joey: "You did what?"

Evan: "Yeah, this guy played well and beat me.

Joey: "Nawwhhh man, you blew it."

These types of conversations were commonplace. Unfortunately, I did not have the experiential background in knowing how to handle not being the best at something. I was a natural sportsman; but in sports, players are only taught how to win, not how to lose. Golf's stiff competition led me to develop some self-esteem issues to the point which I no longer felt the urge to compete and in turn, withdrew from competing in the state tournament. My coach informed me about how I was letting the entire team down by my selfish choice and that I would no longer be on the team if that was my decision. I stood by my decision, as my gut inkling was that I did not want to do it anymore. Something did not feel right.

Night

Most evenings were spent doing pleasurable things like relaxing, watching television, playing video games, reading on the Internet, or even talking on the phone. Just before sunset, I would often chip some golf balls on the miniature hole that I made in the backyard. I stuck a flagpole with a cup near the rear of the yard and spent numerous hours perfecting my short game with my wedges. Music was another outlet for me, as burning mixed CDs was particularly enjoyable. Again, little if any time was allotted towards academia. It was as if school and outside-school were completely different worlds without any overlap. I knew that my genetic blessings would allow me to pass and do fairly well throughout school without much effort. After all, I made it this far without much fortitude. Doing reasonably well was satisfactory by my standards.

Weekends were almost entirely spent with my girlfriend, Jenny Longman. I began dating her at the age of 16 and we continued our steady relationship for approximately three years. No one in either of our families had any objection because we seemed like two youngsters in love. My grandfather did inform me regularly though that I should date around before settling down with just one female. He said that I was too young for a committed relationship, and that an older woman was likely more experienced in various aspects of life. I did not want to hear what he had to say though, so I did not listen. Besides, what did he know? My circumstances were not the same as when he was an adolescent nor as those he had experienced in his 60 years of life. That was my reasoning for not wanting to believe him when I knew he was correct. It is funny how individuals need to learn from their own mistakes rather than learning from our elders and their advice.

Being younger than her, I had additional restrictions and curfews in comparison. It was terrible. Why did my father have to be so unreasonable? After all, I was virtually an all-around saint. Ok, so maybe not, but it was still overburdening to my 16-year-old body. Having to be home by 10:30PM or 11:00PM, I conjured ways to challenge Newton's theories of space and time. I could stretch the amount of time spent at Jenny's house by simply elevating the speed at which I drove home—a very simple, but ingenious method in which I utilized again and again. While still staying within an approximate measure of the speed limit (below twice the legal limit), I generally drove home, arriving on the minute of my curfew. Living life on the edge was the only way I knew. Doing whatever to get what I wanted was what life was all about. After all, I could almost always design a scheme to get out of consequences that I should have received at school or home. I did not particularly care what others thought about me; I was going to do what I wanted, when I wanted, and did not want to hear otherwise. As a teenager and adolescent, my world was the world. Everything that happened had better be in relation to making me happy; otherwise, I was not that concerned with it. This lifestyle was just fine . . . at least on the surface.

There are many other instances representative of being a slacker and self-centered youngster, but that is not the central premise of this composition. This was a depiction of my nonchalant, clueless, and considerably selfish lifestyle that I led prior to undergoing a life-altering event. Looking back on my foolish behavior as a 16-year-old boy, I feel ashamed for many of the actions and attitudes I regularly demonstrated. Still, I firmly believe that *ALL* children, adolescents, and adults are good at heart; they just do what they think they need to in order to feel good, fit in, survive, and/or stay sane.

Chapter 2:

I Have What?

Entering my junior year of high school, I had the world at my fingertips. Anything I wanted was attainable. From athletics to academics, I was blessed with opportunities that allowed me to achieve whatever was pleasing. Being competitive and sports-oriented throughout my childhood and adolescence, I remained in high physical fitness and conditioning without becoming injured except for a broken finger or two. Suddenly the tide began to shift and unlike before, I began to notice that my health was in decline. During the week of final examinations as a junior in high school, I arrived home and headed directly to bed each day. For the next couple of days, I rested more than normal as a method of trying to recuperate. Sleep had a tremendous effect on my body generally. When I obtained ample amounts, I felt great; on the other hand, when I slept little to none, I felt miserable. Obtaining sleep is sometimes cherished while undervalued at other times by many adolescents.

No dinner, no telephone calls, or playing golf. My favorite activities did not even enter into my mind. It felt as if there was no choice. My fatigue was becoming deeper than ever before experienced. Resting was one thing, but going to sleep for the night at 4:00PM in the afternoon was something entirely different. Arriving home each day, I was so tired and totally exhausted. It felt as if I had not slept for even an hour the previous night, even though I had slept over 12 hours for numerous nights consecutively. Perhaps, I was getting too much sleep, or even being too active at school. There were plenty of after-school activities that comprised durations of my time, however, the last couple of weeks of the semester were dedicated strictly to academics. Plus, Baton Rouge Magnet High School, much like other high schools, refrained from holding most of its activities near or during final examinations. Something had to be an underlying problem, but what? The year was coming to a culmination. Clearly there was no time to be sick, depressed, or whatever else that was wrong with me. It was a time to buckle down, focus, and prepare to celebrate another successful year.

Yet, my health concerns were persisting and intensifying in some ways. I had also developed a cough that would not go away. My parents drew upon their prior knowledge and experience of recognizing common infections and sicknesses within their children based on symptomatic feelings. They thought that my tiredness, weakness, loss of appetite, and fever were signs pointing to possibly having a virus like mononucleosis. Then again, the cough could be as a result of bronchitis or some type of respiratory infection. Once before my brother had acquired mononucleosis and I distinctly recalled him lying in bed for days on end. His sickness lasted for two to three weeks, so I supposed that it was a real possibility based on how I was feeling the entire week. My only other complaint was that I could not take in a deep breath of air when lying on my back or stomach, almost as if I were restricted from doing so somehow. As someone who moves around throughout the night, it took me awhile before getting comfortable most nights to fall asleep. That is how I noticed the breathing restriction. Enough was enough; my mother and father decided that it was time to go to the doctor. I was glad to go to my primary-care physician, a Doctor of Internal Medicine, in hopes of providing me with some relief from my ongoing distress.

In the doctor's examination room, Dr. Kawji began conducting typical checks for signs of infection—checking my ears, nose, throat, eyes, lymph nodes, and listening to my lungs. Then, he said that he also needed a urine sample to analyze. Oh, ok, just another step in the sequence of workup. Vital signs, lymph nodes, blood analysis, and urine. Wait a second . . . what? I looked at my mother; our eyes met as she tried to look down. If the doctor was asking for a urine sample, my parents must have set it up. They were trying to secretly have me drug tested to rule out other potential causes of my symptoms. Being somewhat cognizant, I realized what they were doing and happily agreed to supply a sample in the stupid cup to dispel their ridiculous hypothesis of drug use. How dare they question if I were using drugs. The thought perturbed me to the nth degree. After handing over my urine, I remembered that I had failed to inform the doctor about the difficulty I was having breathing in deeply, so I mentioned that symptom as well. He listened to my chest again, and ordered that an X-Ray be taken of my chest as a precautionary measure. Finally, some blood work was drawn for a complete blood cell (CBC) count, which is a panel of screening tests.

Sitting on the doctor's examination table, with my feet swaying front to back, my mother and I waited. It was no different than any other doctor visit, minus the drug testing anyway. Minutes went by and the doctor finally came back with the X-ray films. He posted them on the viewing machines, pointing out his findings.

Directing my attentive and anxious eyes at a massive grey area, he said, "This mass is what is constricting your ability to breathe regularly." It looked quite large to my uneducated eyes and after inquiring about its size, I was informed it was the size of my fist. "You need to see our head oncologist, Dr. Schwartz." This tumor was a mediastinal mass wrapped around a portion of my lungs and heart. Even a 16 year old knew that this was far from good news.

The next step in the process of finding out what in the world was in my chest involved more testing and waiting. Taking some MRIs would provide more accurate information from which diagnostic decisions could be made. A few days later, the images were taken at an imaging specialty clinic and then, it was time to see the oncologist. With my father, mother, and brother with me, we brought X-rays and MRIs into Dr. Schwartz's clinical office. He entered the room, introduced himself, and got right to the point. He turned out the lights and placed various images on two sides of the room depicting the mass in my chest. "You have cancer," said Dr. Schwartz. Did I just hear him correctly . . . I have what? "We need to conduct a biopsy to be certain of the specific diagnosis." Of course, my mother began to freak out hysterically. "Oh, my baby, not my baby," she voiced while sobbing. Meanwhile, my brother wrote down everything the doctor said, using his matter of fact/let's get down to business personality. My father and I listened, while trying to wrap our minds around this announcement. Time stood still for that moment. We had not yet begun to envision how this would soon change all of our lives.

While trying to schedule a biopsy as soon as possible, there were millions of thoughts, questions, and concerns popping in my head continuously—most of which did not receive answers because everything was happening so quickly. Just days before, I was at school laughing and then, doctors would be performing a biopsy of the mediastinal mass in my chest. The head of the oncology department believed that it was likely Hodgkin's Disease based on its proximity, its characteristics, and his 20-something years of experience.

To my knowledge no one in my immediate or distant family had ever been diagnosed with cancer. Questions, hundreds of them, began clouding our minds. Still, the first order of business was finalizing the date as soon as possible for the biopsy to determine what type of cancer was inside my body. As anyone who has ever been to the doctor knows firsthand, scheduling an appointment, let alone a surgery, can be difficult and greatly delayed from one's preferred date. There was no time to argue with nurses and receptionists; my biopsy had to take place immediately. Yet, the surgeon at Our Lake of the Lake Hospital in Baton Rouge, Louisiana, was going on vacation in four days (the end of the week) and his schedule was full leading up to his retreat. Through my father's persistence and pushiness, as well as an oncologist's leadership role in the area, the biopsy was set up for that Friday. It is strange how openings can arise out of thin air, if you know the right people, raise enough hell, or a mixture of the two like my father had thankfully done.

Informing my friends about having cancer was no easy task. There was no easy way to prepare them for the shock, so I used the same method as Dr. Schwartz. "I have cancer" was just as hard to utter to others as it was to accept hearing it. As much as my friends were in disbelief, I could not readily ease their nerves since I did not know much about it myself. The diagnosis was unclear, treatment plans were not known, and I did not know whether I would be around to return to school the following year. So I did the only thing

I could at that time, I prepared myself for the upcoming surgery in a few days.

The biopsy was necessary, but waking up to having an endotracheal tube in my throat was not pleasant. Apparently, there were complications keeping my blood pressure high enough and it was necessary to hook me up to a ventilator. Not having the ability to breathe is scary when awakening from slumber. I began going berserk signaling to the nurses and doctor that they must remove the trachea so I could breathe. It sounded more like, "(pointing to my throat) mmmhhh . . . mhhhhhh." Yet, they continually reassured me to relax and that it was necessary for it to remain, where it occupied my entire airway. Well, there is only so long before one will go mad when others are preventing his body from trying to breathe! As I continued to cause a scene, they communicated with one another agreeing that they needed to pull it out. I could not believe how ridiculous it seemed at the time . . . I had been telling them for what it seemed like a minute or two. It felt like someone had a pillow over my face. Calming down was an impossibility.

Meanwhile, my father stayed diligent, gathering as much information about cancer treatments for Hodgkin's disease as he could. The oncologist, Dr. Schwartz, recommended that I start a treatment protocol there at the same hospital where my biopsy was conducted. This particular treatment involved rounds of chemotherapy and radiation in monthly regiments for about six months. Using this protocol he would reexamine the progression or decline of the cancer in my body periodically. This was the best oncology hospital in the city, but it was not tailored for pediatric patients. Was there anything particular about pediatric oncology? I really did not know. More information was necessary to make an informed decision, but time was of the essence.

Since others suggested that I see someone who specialized in pediatric oncology, we inquired about other options. Pam Trahan, a friend of the family, stayed in regular communication with my father because her son had just completed chemotherapy treatment at an affiliate clinic of St. Jude Children's Research Hospital, next door to the Our Lady of the Lake Hospital in Baton Rouge, Louisiana. She claimed that they were without question the best and that I needed to see Dr. Sheila Moore without delay. My father called her and within minutes of initially speaking with her, she informed my father, "Your child will be cured at St. Jude." Wow. Those were powerful and moving words that brought tears to his eyes. This woman who we had not even met made this bold statement, when the other oncologist stated that my treatment would begin and he would check its' progress periodically. They seemed to be completely different in their confidence levels of their treatment plans. Before ever meeting me, Dr. Sheila Moore's foresight was without question and circumstance. My father made an appointment for me to see her later that day.

Everything was happening so fast. Two hours after getting off a ventilator because of surgery complications at the so-called best hospital in Baton Rouge, I walked to the St. Jude Affiliate Clinic next door. One nurse at St. Jude later commented to me that it was a miracle in itself that I was walking around in the clinic; she had never seen someone so alert and active after just getting off life support. Upon our arrival, my father provided all the medical documents including the X-rays and the MRIs on CD. Dr. Sheila Moore informed me that it was crucial for me to go to Memphis, Tennessee as quickly as possible for a stay of about 10 days. Doctors would begin the process of identifying and treating my illness.

Just as concerns about my health were escalating, I felt some relief in learning my cancer could be treated at St. Jude Children's Research Hospital in 10 days. That duration did not sound too long. Besides, letting them treat my illness now would allow me to be back home so I could get my life back to normal—spending the rest of the summer with my friends. Since Dr. Moore was highly recommended, I took her advice and proceeded to prepare for my brief stint in downtown Memphis, Tennessee. The sooner I left, the better chances I had of surviving. So the next day, we packed and drove to St. Jude Children's Research Hospital without a clue.

One minor complication remained—health insurance. In Baton Rouge, Louisiana, I was still under my father's HMO plan through his employer, a major chemical plant in the area. There were only two oncologists' clinics within my physician network: J. Schwartz, the man with whom I had already seen, and one other. Dad told Schwartz that we were going to St. Jude. The doctor began an ominous speech about how we must not understand that if we go outside the network, we would be 100 percent responsible for all costs associated with medical coverage. This announcement was merely a reiteration of what we already understood. Again, my father was not going to take these restrictions without fighting for the best

opportunity for my well-being.

When inquiring up the chain with Dr. Chaissant, the medical

administrator in the Baton Rouge Stanocola Branch, he repeated

what Dr. Schwartz had already stated. The head of the Ochsner

Group, the company through which I held health insurance, was

located in Metairie, LA. They assigned a date two weeks later at

2:00PM in the afternoon and a phone number. The phone conference

consisted of an allotment of time in minutes as follows: 20-20-20. A

lawyer, physician, counselor, administrator, and another (5 in all)

spoke for approximately 20 minutes from the Ochsner group. Then,

Dr. John Torrey Sandlund, MD., who would be my primary

oncologist at St. Jude Children's Research Hospital, and my father

were granted 20 minutes for talking time followed by a 20-minute

rebuttal. The board explained several factors as to why being treated

in Baton Rouge was a practical option. I was already seeing Dr.

Schwartz and received a diagnosis from his office. He felt that he

could properly treat me. If we were not satisfied with the results, we

could always go to a pediatric oncologist in New Orleans as long as

the doctor remained in network. Yet, they reiterated that Dr.

Schwartz could do an adequate job. My father felt uncomfortable with me receiving treatments with Schwartz because he mainly dealt with adult patients and his methods for treating pediatric patients consisted of using smaller doses of the same therapies. Not to mention, by that time, I had already discovered that Schwartz had misdiagnosed the cancer in my body. Why would he be suitable for treating an illness he failed to properly diagnose?

Dr. Sandlund declared that the preliminary diagnosis was bogus. He voiced how I had just begun treatment at St. Jude Children's Research Hospital that included high-dose chemotherapy specifically targeting T-Cell lymphoma. This included a number of drugs that I would not have received in Baton Rouge. He urged the medical review board saying, "These drugs are needed and necessary, critical for his survival in this life-threatening time with our researched treatment programs."

The board reached their decision only five minutes later. They contended that I would only be covered to receive medical care locally. Dr. Sandlund and my father rebutted for at least 10 more minutes, but to no avail. My father continued, "You cannot and will not put a price on my son's life." The decision was steadfast and there would be no coverage outside the network. My father decided to change his insurance policy as soon as possible; yet, it was not until the first of every year that changes to his renewals were permitted. Until that date, St. Jude Children's Research Hospital covered all costs associated with my cancer treatment. Furthering his fight for justice, my dad filed a petition at the home office of Ochsner in Baton Rouge. No notification or consideration was ever given to his request.

Meanwhile, on the opposite side of the spectrum of the medical world, St. Jude Children's Research Hospital continues to lead the world in pediatric oncology, relying solely upon charitable donations from wonderful individuals and corporations. Through these blessings, my expenses were fully paid during the six months prior to our change of insurance policies. St. Jude Children's Research Hospital continues to this day to pay all costs associated with the treatment of patients who cannot afford or whose insurance plans refuse to cover the costs, because they are not a business; they are a team housed in a facility in which children are healed and where life is valued more than the dollar.

Although it was settled that I would be going to Memphis, TN for several days, I was still in disbelief. Yes, I was sick. I had also seen the X-rays and MRIs with my own eyes, and even heard doctors say that I had cancer. I figured though that somehow, someway there must have been some type of mistake. How could a fun-loving and seemingly healthy 16 year old develop cancer? Besides, I could not possibly have cancer. I was invincible. As golf team captain and social class clown, I had too much going for me. These thoughts rushed through my head like it were the final moment of my life. I had not even begun to comprehend what having cancer would entail. Those three words (you have cancer) were instantly etched into my mind forever. Engaging in discourse with concerned friends and family was difficult due to so many uncertainties. How did you acquire cancer? Was it hereditary? What is your likelihood of surviving this disease? These were good questions; I just did not have the answers.

I began to realize that my life would never be the same. Everything was somehow different now. One day I was enjoying joking with my classmates at lunch; the next I had to pack some clothes and drive to St. Jude Children's Research Hospital in

Memphis, Tennessee. Would my health-related problems really be cured within 10 days? Most of the time when I thought of cancer, elderly people who were already on their deathbed came to mind. My ignorance was quickly diminishing, as I was in the hot seat. I did not know what the word cancer even meant—something to do with cells going haywire in the body. I just knew that thousands of people die from various forms of cancer each year. Many of whom did something in their lifetime to contribute to their development of the cancer. Was this why I had developed cancer? Had I somehow placed my body in harm's way through exposure to chemicals, sanitation practices, or engaging in sexual intercourse for the first time only months earlier? I began backtracking through all of my childhood and adolescence to resolve my anxiety about encounters that could have been contributing factors. Reflecting on one's life in a few minutes was entirely difficult as it forced the brain to encapsulate everything memorable and toss out the rest. As a result, I recalled a few instances where my body could have been exposed to harmful substances.

The first memory was related to the proximity of my residence to Dawson's Creek in Baton Rouge, Louisiana. My friends and I could be found playing in the woods, building forts, climbing trees, and fishing. Fishing was enjoyable. We never kept any of the fish, especially since they were mostly gar fish. About every five years or so, we noticed fish kills, where every living species including gar, tarp, catfish, bass, brim, turtles, and snakes could be found floating or on the banks of the creek. These fish kills were infrequent, but they were directly behind my house, and possibly a sign that a substance in large quantities had been dumped in the creek. It was interesting though that this was going on within 50 yards of my house. Moreover, my birthplace is informally known as Cancer Alley. Some anecdotal evidence purports that this region (along the Mississippi River from Baton Rouge to New Orleans) has a higher preponderance of cancer diagnoses per capita than most other places in the United States.

Other than those startling recollections, there were only a handful of other possibilities. Just months prior to my diagnosis, I was working in a sometimes unsanitary environment preparing frozen summertime treats for the locals. Additionally, there were hundreds of times I dealt with gasoline doing yard work and other jobs growing up. Yet, I decided that none of these instances with carcinogenic substances were likely to have accounted for the abnormal and unexplained development of cancer. I failed to reach a breakthrough of any kind. The cause of my cancer remained unknown and will likely remain unknown for some time. One thing though was certain—what was supposed to be a 10 days of tests and treatment turned into a life-changing two and one-half years.

Chapter 3:

From the Suburbs to Downtown

After driving 380 miles northeastward from Baton Rouge, my father, mother, brother, and I arrived in Memphis, where we were greeted at the hospital gate. The attendant was polite, asking for my dad's license information and plate number. As the man was speaking with my father, I started thinking about why a hospital would have a 10-foot fence surrounding it. Fences are constructed for one of two reasons: to keep people contained or to keep others out. Either way, it was quite peculiar. I remembered that as we drove into the city, the hospital was located directly in the downtown region of the city. Having never before visited the great city of Memphis, my first visit was an eye-opening experience. All I knew about the city is that it was home to St. Jude, the University of Memphis, Rhodes College, the Memphis Grizzlies National Basketball Association (NBA) team, and Graceland.

Gaining entry into the hospital facility was carefully restricted with guards and at least two security points before actually going into the hospital. Proceeding through the first check point, we followed the guard's directions before heading into the underground parking garage. After entering the doors of the hospital, I heeded information displayed on wall signs that directed me towards the clinical section in which I would be seen. A-Clinic was dedicated to the research and treatment of leukemias and lymphomas. Two doctors, Drs. Pui and Sandlund, co-led this clinic where they acted as both the clinical doctors for every patient at St. Jude who had either leukemia or lymphoma, and simultaneously led hundreds of researchers at the hospital, other hospitals, pharmaceutical corporations, and programs abroad. These two men not only collaborated in the research of the effectiveness of chemotherapy regimens but also acted as caring, loving, and mindful doctors who did everything for their patients. In the rare instances of hospital workers not treating one of their patients with utmost consideration or respect, they would be personally summoned by these doctors.

I arrived at the hospital on a Saturday afternoon, and there were three nurses who were working in the medicine room. They seemed fairly laid back and not overly busy. There were hospital beds hugging three sides of the room. I began to survey the room, scanning for similarities and differences to other hospital rooms. Never before had I been in a medicine room, whatever that meant.

53

The term medicine room sounded like a place where a pharmacist would hand patients some pills to take. Why was there this large room with beds everywhere? The white walls, white beds, white sheets, and white-colored equipment made for an eerie feeling. One male nurse approached, introducing himself as Stan. He welcomed us to St. Jude. Having briefly inquired as to our needs, I updated him of our arrival from Baton Rouge, Louisiana and that we would be staying for the next 10 days. Typing my information into their systems, he found detailed information as to what types of lab work were to be conducted. Stan directed us to an individual room where he would meet us shortly. In the room, my brother and I sat on the available chairs while my father stood and my mother sat on the floor against one of the walls. Something did not make sense to me. I had already gone through the process of doing blood work in Baton Rouge. Why did I have to get more here? Even so, it did not cause any legitimate concern. A little bit of lab work never killed anyone. Well, that's what I thought before Stan wheeled out the tray.

Stan pushed a tray containing an arsenal of instruments like he was preparing for surgery or perhaps even a genetic research experiment. There were 10 small blood vials, 7 larger ones, tubing all over, tourniquets, and needles of every size, I started questioning whether I was in the right place. Was this a hospital where healing takes place, or a torture chamber where people undergo undue pain? I had seen movies that included scenes like this, and I was not interested in participating in any ordeal leading to those gory outcomes. Stan tried to ease my nerves by saying that it would not be so bad. I figured it was easier for the one drawing the blood to make such a comment. He began just as any nurse would: putting the tourniquet over my bicep, telling me to make a fist, and starting to pluck the veins in my mid-arm. "Oh, that's a hose right there," said Stan, referring to the easiness to which he could stick one vein in particular. I had no qualms about needles or having blood drawn; it was the voluminous supply of tools and tubules that seemed daunting. As Stan went from one to the next, time passed by extremely slowly. It was as if it took him forever to finish his blood thievery. Eventually, I began feeling light-headed. Near the end of the blood withdrawal, my mother started passing out as she saw my eyes spinning. Even my brother was not feeling too well, having seen what effect it had on me. I longed for the whole damn blood work thing to be over. Finally, it concluded. Thank God, that was the end of my trouble for that day. "Whew . . . that was crazy," I thought. I did not know it at the time, but in hindsight, it was child's play. Much harder battles were faced on a daily basis for a much longer duration than the expected 10 days in Memphis.

Again, Stan, my nurse, was calm, polite, and extremely helpful in directing me to where I needed to go. He handed me a Monday schedule that included an order of events for my first full-fledged hospital visit. It had a long list of times and places; most of which I knew nothing about. Stan said the only other thing I needed to do was to go back to the receptionist in the front foyer to pick up my hotel and meal vouchers. Really? St. Jude was not only going to not only pay for my family to stay in Memphis at a hotel, but also pay for our meals. How was this possible? No other hospitals I had ever been to followed this procedure. But hey, I was not going to complain.

I approached the front desk again, speaking with the same woman who had already placed an identification wrist bracelet on me. This woman was also friendly, just like Stan and the gate attendant. From the very beginning, just about every person affiliated with the hospital was amiable. She handed me a hotel voucher for the La Quinta Inn and Suites in midtown Memphis. Since my father was driving, I let him handle the driving directions aspect of the conversation with the receptionist. Then, meal tickets were given. She explained that at the time St. Jude provided each patient 6 dollars for breakfast, 8 dollars for lunch, and 10 dollars for dinner. My father did not feel the need to take the meal tickets, because we believed that charity was for those less fortunate. Since we were not living paycheck to paycheck, there was not a need. The woman recommended that we take them anyway and so, we did reluctantly. Whether we would use them could be decided at a later time. Thanking her for her kindness and helpfulness, we departed the foyer, headed back down to the parking garage, and drove away from the hospital towards our hotel for some much needed rest and relaxation.

During the hospital visit, our hunger grew. We were famished from the six-hour drive and introductory lab work at St. Jude. On the way to the hotel, we grabbed some food at a local hamburger joint, which was exactly what everyone needed to regain some much needed energy. I decided on a huge hamburger, large fries, and a lemon-lime beverage; it was just what the doctor ordered. After eating the scrumptious meal, we drove around the corner to check in at our hotel. Representatives of St. Jude had already reserved our stay at the facility, which was very thoughtful and allowed us to focus on our own concerns.

Half-way unpacking took about 30 minutes. Meanwhile, a couple of us took showers. After all, there was nothing worse than not showering after being cramped in a vehicle most of the day. Just as the day was beginning to wind down, we clicked on the television set to see what types of channels this hotel received. There were quite a few from which to choose. Eventually my mother decided to watch the movie, *The Negotiator*, on HBO. I sprawled out on the bed, trying to get comfortable with all that ran through my mind like being in an unfamiliar hotel of a new city, going to a new hospital, and a newfound discovery of an illness. About 20 minutes into the motion picture, we got a rude awakening. BOOM! The door to our room flew open, as it was busted in by a man. Ahhhh! We were scared for our lives. A man slammed the door open with his shoulder and stood in our room. Was he a crack fiend looking for money, or possibly a criminal looking to steal our belongings? Before we could even say, "What the hell?," the man said, "I'm security. I am just doing my nightly door checks. Your door was unlocked." Each of us had a puzzled look on our face, but did not say anything to the man. He shut the door and left. One second, we were watching the movie, and then our door was slammed in by a stranger whose nametag read, Chester. Within a total of five seconds, things were back to normal. We never saw this individual again. All of us sat up looking at one another, commenting how that was the strangest thing we had ever witnessed. Our door was not wide open, but merely unlocked. Thank God, we were not changing clothes or anything. From that moment, we had a new opinion of the hotel, making it our first and last stay. If we were to survive and flourish in Memphis, we had to toughen up, stay alert, and always be mindful of where we were at all times.

Memories are the foundation from which we proceed in our daily lives. In Memphis, there were several experiences that jostled my way of thinking and seeing the world. The following day after the security guard barged into our hotel room, mom and I relaxed in the room most of the day, knowing that a full-day at the hospital would follow on Monday. For dinner, no one felt like getting dressed up and going to a restaurant so my father and brother decided to drive to a fast-food restaurant nearby to pick up food. We came to the city in my dad's 1990 Acura Legend, so my brother thought it would be an opportune time to continue learning to drive a car equipped with a manual transmission. They departed but failed to return for 40 minutes. Gosh, mom and I asked what in the world took them so long. It marked yet another incident in our first two days in the city of Memphis.

Erich and dad pulled up in the drive-thru of a popular fast-food chain. Naturally, Erich rolled down his window, as they looked at the menu displayed in lights as the sun began to set. Erich looked at my dad, asking what he thought they should order. Simultaneous to Erich's turning of his head towards the passenger side of the vehicle, a man jumped out from the bushes underneath the menu, stuck his head almost entirely inside the vehicle stating, "Y'all can give me five dollars?" Ahh, Erich began panicking, as dad yelled, "Get us the hell out of here." Stepping into action, Erich floored the pedal, forgetting it also required him to release his foot from the clutch pedal. Vrrrooooommm! The car went nowhere, as it revved up the rpms considerably. "Whatever you do, just don't let the car die," said Dad. Erich thought for a split-second, used the clutch, and drove the car unintentionally on and over the curb, as the Legend peeled out of the drive-thru line while bucking rapidly from Erich's letting off the clutch too soon. Mom and I were in disbelief, and did the only thing we knew how at that point—we laughed. "That is crazy," I said. After the incident at the drive-thru, they went to another place to grab some burgers before coming back to the hotel. And so, our view was becoming more and more ingrained about living and surviving in downtown Memphis. We were not concerned with flourishing; we just wanted to get by, take care of business, and get the heck out of there.

Moving to Memphis was a drastic change—living downtown, sometimes without personal transportation, and in a community-living facility. Being 380 miles away from home also prevented me from doing some of the simple things in my life that I had grown to love. Going to a friend's house or playing golf after school were not feasible anymore. As senseless as that may seem, what I had taken for granted was no longer possible. In an instant, my life changed; in two and one-half years, my life changed every single day. Getting cancer and partaking in the excruciating pain and agony of chemotherapy each and every week defined those aspects of my life that were important and those that were not. I was no longer worried about petty aspects of my life. Nothing else really mattered. What actually mattered was staying alive and fighting for a future, free of pain, suffering, and endless days in which only sleep numbed my feeble body. I regularly propositioned doctors to put me into an induced coma for the two and one-half years and then wake me up when they were done torturing my mind and body. My attempts failed; perhaps, the doctors made the correct decision. At the time, it did not seem that way though. It is sometimes through agony and strife that one can appreciate the blessing of life.

Chapter 4:

A Realization

WHY? Anyone can selfishly and continually ask questions about why he/she was chosen to have cancer, but it is not a worthwhile endeavor. In many instances like mine, there was not a specific cause identified by the doctors. So naturally I began to wonder and reflect on all my life experiences trying to identify circumstances and environmental encounters that could have contributed to my development of cancer. There had to be a reason why I was afflicted with cancer and no one else around me was.

Beyond having a large amount of blood work performed two days earlier, I learned that I was misdiagnosed in Baton Rouge, LA. Misdiagnosed . . . that is ridiculous. Not only did Dr. Schwartz, the oncologist in Baton Rouge and second in charge at the *best* hospital in the city, misdiagnose me but he also suggested a protocol for treatment at a local clinic that was drastically different from that of the one St. Jude suggested for me to begin. Instead of having Hodgkin's disease, I was diagnosed, accurately this time, with Stage III non-Hodgkin's Lymphoblastic Lymphoma (NHL) (Thymus Cell). Having quickly researched various treatment programs at St.

Jude, the only difference that I knew at the time was that Hodgkin's disease had an accompanied chemotherapy protocol lasting nine months while the one for NHL was two and one-half years. Yay, now I had a cancerous disease that had a lower survival rate (70%) and it took more than one and one-half additional years to complete. Each day became more difficult and thus, tensions continued to rise as well.

What I had was of serious concern. In 1999, the survival rate for patients with non-Hodgkin's lymphoma was 70% at St. Jude Children's Research Hospital. Patients cared for in other hospital facilities varied in their cure rates, not that it mattered because I was not going to play Russian roulette with my life. I went to the best facility in the world for pediatric oncology.

Just 40 years previously (1959), NHL patients only had a 4% survival rate. Just 10 years after my diagnosis (2009), the cancer survival rate had already increased to 85%. Astounding breakthroughs in science have allowed thousands of patients to stay alive. Still, what if I were in that 30% who did not survive? My life and future existence was uncertain. I might not live through this treatment, so was it really worth going through all that pain and suffering that people spoke of regarding chemotherapy? Even if I were cured from NHL with the treatment program, there was a 30% chance that cancer would reoccur within five years of being in remission. It sounded like just the kind of never-ending battle of uncertainty that did not settle easily with a control freak like me.

Being a curious teenager, I wanted to learn more about my disease. Having access to the Internet, I read as many articles as I could find on the subject. I did not realize how rare my form of cancer was for someone my age. One day while my mother was preparing a meal at the Ronald McDonald House, I found a book that detailed statistical information about various cancers including NHL. I read that the likelihood that a male aged 14-19 years old would acquire NHL was 7:1,000,000. Wow! Only seven in a million boys my age were diagnosed with the same type of cancer. I guess that meant that I was in a select crowd, but unlike most parts of life, there was no trophy for this select few.

Friends, family, and acquaintances heard news of my illness within the first several weeks of my diagnosis. Just as I was unfamiliar with the disease, so were they. One friend, Joseph Bergeron, M.D., did not know what to think. He and I were best buddies in high school and this period of time was well before he became a medical doctor. Upon hearing of my diagnosis, Joey thought that non-Hodgkin's lymphoma signified that it was non-malignant. As a result, he never considered that my life was in jeopardy. This case in point serves as an indicator that the terminology within the specialized field of medicine is foreign to laymen. The lack of transparency creates a barrier in communication and understanding between physicians and patients. It became my mission to learn more than just superficial facts about my disease to prevent my continued ignorance.

Non-Hodgkin's lymphomas originate in the lymphatic system where tumors develop from lymphocytes—types of white blood cells. The specific type that I was diagnosed with, T-cell lymphoma, represents less than 15% of non-Hodgkin's lymphomas in the United States. According to the American Cancer Society (2009):

> It often starts in the thymus gland (where T cells are made) and can develop into a large tumor in the mediastinum (the area around the heart and behind the breast bone). This can cause trouble breathing if it presses on the windpipe (trachea)

leading into the lungs. It can also block the superior vena cava (the large vein that returns blood to the heart from the arms and head), which can cause the arms and face to swell. This lymphoma is fast-growing, but if it hasn't spread to the bone marrow when it is first diagnosed, the chances of being cured with chemotherapy are quite good. Once it is in the bone marrow, only about 40%-50% of patients can be cured.

Worldwide, it is common practice to use the Ann Arbor Staging System to describe the spread of NHL in adults. In my situation, doctors at St. Jude used the same staging so as to minimize any confusion when sharing and disseminating information pertaining to my case. There are four stages described with Roman numerals I-IV (1-4).

Stage I—   indicates that the lymphoma is only located in one specific region,

or

the cancer is only found in one single organ outside the lymph system

Stage II—   lymphoma is in 2 or more groups of lymph nodes on the same side of the diaphragm, *or*

the lymphoma extends locally from a single group of lymph nodes into a nearby organ

Stage III—   lymphoma is found in lymph node areas on both sides of the diaphragm, *or*

the cancer may have extended into an area or organ next to the lymph nodes, into the spleen, or both

Stage IV—   lymphoma has spread outside of the lymph system into an organ not next to the involved node, *or*

the lymphoma has spread to the bone marrow, liver, brain, spinal cord, or the pleura (thin lining of the lungs)

The etiology or cause of non-Hodgkin's lymphoma (NHL) is not known. It is not possible to spread or become infected with NHL from contact with someone who has it. Neither alcohol consumption nor injury has been linked with the onset of NHL. Some common risk factors associated with the development of non-Hodgkin's lymphoma include having a weak immune system, viral infections, and environmental considerations that include working with or touching hazardous/toxic materials. The likelihood of onset increases with age and occurs more frequently in males.

According to my father, my grandfather (Paw Paw) maintained a simplistic view about what causes cancer. His perspective closely matched mine which revolves around the idea of genes turning on and off. Paw Paw told my dad that everybody has it in them; in some people, a switch is turned on which allows the cancer to begin growing. Although this belief seemed rather odd at the time, it is similar to genetic investigations that track the origins of rapid cell division and growth today.

Even though it is natural to question why someone has developed cancer, one needs to understand that it is not a matter of being chosen to bear the burden. I had to keep in mind that sometimes bad things happen to good people. Those cells grew out of control (rapidly dividing); mutations are a naturally-occurring part of life. Put quite simply—the stress that I put on myself at 16 years old probably increased the degree to which my body was susceptible to getting ill. Although stress does not solve problems, it was harder to understand when I was young, self-centered, and often depressed about something as irrelevant as not getting my way on a certain

69

matter. If only I could have had 60 years of wisdom, a 16-year-old's energy, and a newborn's joyful spirit, I would have had a well-rounded outlook on day-to-day life.

What is God's role in all of this?

Some folks are steadfast believers that life is already predetermined before they are even born. But if this were true, why did God give us free will to act, make choices, and the ability to think for ourselves? Others proclaim that everything happens for a reason. But there is no reasoning involved when innocent children develop cancer. There is no reason when someone's daughter dies from cancer at the age of 12. There is no reason when a teenager dies of cancer leaving both siblings and parents to mourn for their loss.

Many events, circumstances, and tribulations are not caused or directed by the hand of God, but instead are a result in part of the world in which we live. Our God is not a vengeful king, but a loving Father, who gave us the potential and guiding words to live justly. God did not set out to punish people on earth for whatever types of sins they have committed. Sometimes, bad things just happen.

On a recent yearly checkup trip to St. Jude, I was transported from the hospital to the airport with several other families after my full day of MRIs and scans. Visiting with the other patients is one of my favorite activities because there is so much to be learned from these children. Their perspectives on life are remarkable. One passenger just learned that she had some brain tumors reappear in the form of a different type of cancer. This 11-year-old girl, Cindy, was also legally blind and extra talkative. She spoke to her friend on a cellular phone about how she would have to come back to Memphis next week to begin some radiation and chemotherapy. Meanwhile, her mother sobbed and visibly showed signs of depression over the recent discovery. Cindy explained that her disease was rare and that the experimental treatment program would be highly individualized. And then, one of her comments made me raise my eyebrows and think. She said, "Well, it's just one more thing . . . it's not like I haven't done it before, and I know that God would never give me more than I can handle, so I'm not worried about it." Perhaps, the world can learn a lot from Cindy. Faith and hope are real.

It took me quite some time and thought to figure this out on my own. Originally, I thought that God was punishing me for being a mischievous troublemaker as an adolescent, as I described in the first chapter. I figured that all of those selfish acts had finally caught up with me. Now they were going to cost me dearly. That was before I came to the realization that God was not actually responsible for any of my suffering. God allows mankind to make their own decisions and live their lives accordingly; he just asks that we make the best of what we have. This is why I will never stop working with and for those who need help like cancer patients. They deserve assistance from those more capable and that is the least we can do to comfort them.

Rather than gripe and complain about it not being fair, all of the focus should turn towards defeating and ridding the body of such a disease. Time is especially of the essence when even minutes of indecisiveness can result in death. The reason behind acquiring cancer is not important; the resolution must be the focal point. Not one iota of energy can be expended elsewhere. Not only does a person have to be concerned about himself, but his entire family and friends must be committed to the cause. I do not know one person who has ever defeated cancer on one's own; a collaborative team effort must be present and in unison for such a battle. Words like battle or war are used to describe bouts with cancer because it is single-handedly hell on earth. No words are fit to describe the feelings that accompany sessions of chemotherapy. Language cannot truly communicate the suffering of battling cancer and undergoing chemotherapy nor can it represent the elation that accompanies daily life afterwards.

Chapter 5:

Initial Changes

After meeting with my oncologist at St. Jude, I was impressed with his apparent intelligence and genuine kindness. He seemed like just the guy for the job. We spoke and he facilitated all of our questions pertaining to the cancer and my future treatment of the disease. When I learned that the treatment was going to include two induction phases and weekly regiments of chemotherapy for two and one-half years, I was anything but thrilled. The shock set in that my life was going to be solely focused on this disease—non-Hodgkin's lymphoma. What followed was the signing of nearly 50 pages of liability documents pertaining to the treatment of my disease as an experimental study. Indeed, this was the leading pediatric cancer institute in the United States, so my reservations were limited. My father and I signed the papers because I was a minor. Even before chemotherapy began, it was suggested to make an outside appointment with a sperm clinic in Memphis. This was no ordinary visit like a blood analysis or profile; this appointment was necessary so that I could store my sperm in case I became infertile. A sick adolescent traveling with his family to a new city and going to store his sperm at a clinic did not exactly make for an idealistic outing.

Just the thought of *doing my business* and then handing it to someone else felt incredibly awkward. With my father's encouragement, I decided that it was in my best interest to store my sperm since possible side effects of chemotherapy I would be receiving included infertility. So Tuesday, my father and I went to the facility, which was located in Northeast Memphis towards Germantown. It looked like a reputable place, resembling any medical doctor's office from the outside of the building. Even inside, it appeared just like any other medical facility. There were receptionists out front and nurses/lab techs in the back directing me where to go. I was sent into a room, where a woman informed me to simply exit the room with the sample when I was finished. That's it? I assumed they felt no more directions were needed. Two thoughts emanated: 1) Jeesh, did I really have to do this in a container with an opening the size of a bottle cap? and 2) The room in which I was standing was very strange. It was way too large, first of all, measuring probably 20 feet wide and 30 feet long. Couches, recliners, and seats littered the room, not to mention dirty magazines, posters, and other pornographic paraphernalia. It resembled lounges where guys would go to drink, watch sporting events, and rant and rave about their significant others . . . like I had seen in movies. Then, I noticed that there were an exuberant number of doors in the room, probably five in all. What if someone came in and caught me in the middle of acquiring a sample? That was plenty enough reason for me to be anxious. And as everyone knows, anxiety and sperm samples do not go hand-in-hand. Nevertheless, I grabbed one of the non-academic pieces of literature to peruse, trying to focus on the task at hand. Where should I sit? Again, there were chairs, couches, recliners, and every other kind of sitting place. How could one be certain that the entire room was sterilized between frequenters to the facility? There was no way in my mind that someone could disinfect the entire room every time, so I decided rather than to take the risk, I would just stand. With that said, I did not produce the most generous sample when I finally achieved completion.

Exiting the room, the lab tech took the container, asking "That's it?" I guess it did not meet her standards. What a hussy. But that was what came out—take it or leave it. I went back to the waiting area with my father, where we sat for about 30 minutes while the sperm was put in a centrifuge before being examined under a 40x microscope. The only reason I know the specifics is because I later re-conducted the study in the confines of a laboratory at Louisiana State University.

The lab technician came out to greet us, telling me that I would be unable to store a sample there because I had no living sperm in my semen sample. "What do you mean, lady?" Before ever beginning chemotherapy, I had a zero sperm count. NOW WHAT? Not only do I have to endure chemotherapy for years, but I cannot ever be a father. It sounded like the worst scenario possible. Thanks a lot for taking my $180 dollars and my only future aspiration in life. How in the hell did my semen already have a zero sperm count? It was not like it was just low and medication could be given to possibly increase the number of living sperm; I had none living at all. Devastation set in, and it has not ceded much even today as I write this memoir 10 years later.

Familial changes

Being in Memphis, Tennessee for 11 weeks during the summer of 1999 created some logistical difficulties for my family. Everyone wanted to be in Memphis with me caring and assisting;

77

however, the real world continued at home. My younger sister, Monica, was only 12 years old. Like any other preteen, she had her own concerns and priorities. My parents, though, informed her via direct and indirect methods that those would have to take a back seat to my needs. Although this was indeed a necessary and justifiable way of looking at the circumstances, she never got to experience three years of her life; instead, she experienced three years of my life. Her kindness was even sometimes underappreciated. The evidence lies in my remembrance of one day after receiving a chemotherapy treatment. I asked Monica if she would get me some cocoa (using a faint, sickly voice). She responded with, "Get it yourself!" Monica claims to this day that she was joking and that it was the only occurrence of not doing everything I asked of her. Further, she says that she retrieved the chocolate milk for me anyway. I frankly do not remember, but I have my doubts.

On the other hand, my brother, Erich, had just completed high school and was in the midst of preparing to move into a college dormitory on the campus of Louisiana State University. He was involved with his first real girlfriend and was head over heels and in the palm of her hand (whip cracks here). His concerns were living it up, working at the local McDonald's for spending money, and planning for his collegiate goals—determining what would be his major, getting a feasible course schedule, and maintaining relationships with others from high school now that they were branching out to universities around the nation. Since he would not be living at home anymore, he and I did not spend nearly as much time together as we had been accustomed. We shared a room for over 10 years. From fights and basketball competitions to impressing teenage babysitters and high school antics, we were best friends. I was losing my brother, my best friend, and my roommate—the person I always knew I could depend on.

The same person with whom I was not spending much time was the same person with whom my friends spent their time. It is true that most of our friends were mutual acquaintances, because I began attending the high school where he had already completed his freshmen year. Thus, I benefitted from his network of friends in terms of transitioning to high school. However, that did not mean that some of those friends and other ones of mine were not dear to me. My greatest friend on earth, Dr. Joseph P. Bergeron, began hanging out with my brother when I was too sick to chill or play golf on the weekends. The telephone rang on many instances and hearing

Joey ask to speak to my brother felt awful. It was true that I could

not voice much at all without feeling completely nauseous, but that

did not mean that my feelings were still not hurt. It was as if the

roles were reversed. Instead of me befriending and growing close to

my brother's friends like Timothy Marchiafava and Ira Register, it

was Erich, my brother, growing closer with Joey. It is beautiful to

see relationships blossom; that is if it does not make you even sicker

to your stomach.

My parents were forced to mend any disputes that had arisen

since their divorce of four years. My mother having since re-married,

had to socialize, cooperate, and live with my father at times in the

Ronald McDonald House. These circumstances were anything but

ideal, but they allowed me to see that they still loved one another and

their children. At the time of my diagnosis and throughout my cancer

treatment, their responsibilities did not disappear like mine; instead,

they held an extra burden of caring for me, since I desperately

needed the assistance.

The summer of 1999 stretched across 380 miles. My family

alternated in taking primary caretaking roles and providing for me.

These rotational shifts began with my father returning home to work four days a week, Tuesday through Friday. Each week, he left from work to drive six hours to Memphis. He not only always provided financially for his family but also comforted his children whenever we needed it for our entire lives; this was no exception. Mom took the primary caretaking role during the week, every week for the first six weeks or so. Returning to Memphis one week with my grandmother, Maw Maw, Mom felt that I could use extended motherly love that always came with a smile. Maw Maw helped Mom with a range of tasks including the cooking duties, which I always appreciated and still do today.

During those two stints in Memphis, the Ronald McDonald House provided us a suitable living arrangement with which to reside. In this community-living environment, my family network instantly extended to many of the other families. Several ones in particular stand out like the Burkins family. These Midwesterners were not accustomed to living in a city of 650,000 people. In fact, their daily rituals of living on a farm, milking the cows, and growing their own food made it difficult to transition towards downtown city life. These compassionate individuals always cooked, having more than enough food for everyone who wanted it. It did not bother me one bit; I was happy to receive the benefit of nourishment. The son, Daniel, was 17 years old. By the time I arrived, he was already showing signs of steroid use with a puffy face and pot belly. He looked like he weighed about 220 pounds; meanwhile, I was about 100 pounds lighter than him. He and I were cancer patients who looked similar in some regards and different in others. Daniel experienced many of the same physical ailments that I did, just months in advance. During his stay, he seemed to remain in good spirits in part because of his loving family, positive motivation, and drive to defeat the cancer and move on to bigger and better opportunities in life. It was hard to see his family leave. My mother and grandmother had grown close to his mother—a calm, polite, and always generous woman.

Not all families were as auspicious during their stay at the Ronald McDonald House. Many children with cancer had single mothers who were still working during their child's chemotherapy treatments. So how does that work? One young child I distinctly remember was named Trey. This fun-spirited seven-year-old boy was always running around the living quarters unsupervised.

Naturally, he was curious when we were in the kitchen, eating area, or the game room. "What ch'all doin?" and "Gimme some" were his favorite expressions. We offered him some of our food when he was around, as he always acted like he was starving. He told us that his mother worked sometimes at night. It was obvious that he did not receive proper parental care, but there was not much we could do about it other than assist him when he hung around us.

Other families were intact when their child was first diagnosed. Soon after moving in the Ronald McDonald House in Memphis, TN, I met the family of the person with whom I grew closest, Seth Strick. His family was from Maryland. Seth's father stayed with him more than his mother because it was difficult for her to be present and watch him each day, plus his father was a business man who could complete some of his duties via the computer. Throughout his stay, I grew very close to his entire family as he and I hung out several times each week and ate together often. He was expected to finish his induction phase before me, but when doctors conducted some imaging scans of his brain, they found additional tumors.

"More tumors!" his dad told us. "That's just great." I think that Seth was not as disappointed as his father. As a matter of fact, Seth appeared relatively calm when he told me that the doctors did not know much about the specific type of cancer that was found. The name evades me years later, but the aftermath was quite memorable. Only a few short weeks later, I was informed by his father that Seth was no longer living. Seth was dead. Memorial services were held back in his hometown of Maryland. The individual with whom I most closely aligned myself did not successfully conquer the cancer in his body. Was this a foreshadowing of what would come for me? I was not comfortable knowing that at any given moment cancer could present itself again and kill me.

A guy from my high school named Josh, who was two years older than me, was also battling brain tumors like my friend Seth. Josh was receiving radiation therapy at St. Jude too. The only reason I knew Josh was from physical education class in high school. We took golf class together and he thought that he was hot stuff. His confident personality clashed with mine. Combined with the notion that I was a sophomore, we did not always act kindly towards one another. It goes to show that trivial details of everyday life often get in the way of those larger issues and matters of the world.

On several occasions, I saw him and his mother when they came to St. Jude every couple of weeks. The more time I spent at St. Jude, the more I realized that I was not alone in my battle with cancer. Thousands of others, younger and older than me, were in similar predicaments. All of my pain was being shared by others. Through conversing and befriending those who were also suffering, it eased the pain with which we felt. It was much easier to speak with cancer patients about my thoughts and feelings than ordinary people—others would not have been able to relate. Lucky them!

After staying at the La Quinta Inn for the first week in Memphis, I was upgraded to the Ronald McDonald House adjacent to the St. Jude Hospital. This living headquarters was built to house patients and their families who were staying in Memphis for more than a few days. Another facility, the Target House, housed patients staying 12 weeks or longer. Nevertheless, the Ronald McDonald House or "the crib" as my family referred to it was home for the next 11 weeks. Our one room luxury suite had two double beds, a foldout chair, and bathroom. Downtown's finest for sure. Still, we tried to make it more like home by putting up a bulletin board where I posted cards and letters I received from people in Louisiana. In addition, my father also brought my own television and computer to the room two weeks later. All sorts of people were sending me calling cards that allowed me to contact my loved ones easily. Monetary sums and toys were other popular gifts. This dormitory style of living also had a shared kitchen and dining room area. Every four families shared a kitchen and pantry area. The mutual dining area provided for convenient interactions amongst the families, not to mention the loud and crazy siblings of cancer patients running amuck through the hallways. Yet, many times I felt too sick to go down to the kitchen to eat. My loving mother babied me continuously, just what I needed at the time, giving me whatever whenever. Still, I did not have that much of an appetite most of the time since I was so sick. That was until I got on Dexamethasone. This drug, if taken for more than a week at a time, has such an overwhelming effect on the body that it is truly unimaginable. Being on Dex, to which it was commonly referred, for three weeks in a row was crazy. All of a sudden I had an appetite that could not be suppressed. Eating did not quench my desire for food. I ate and I ate

86

and I ate, but to no avail. And it wasn't just that I was eating because I felt like it. I had stomach pains so bad that my body was telling me I had to eat. Snacks consisted of two entire bags of Tostitos alongside one jar of cheese dip and one jar of salsa. Within an hour, these were completely annihilated. I remember having a conversation with my mom:

Mom: "What did you do with the chips?"

Evan: "Well, I ate them."

Mom: "I know, but where are the rest?"

Evan: "There is nothing left."

Mom: "Huh, you gotta be kidding me."

From that moment, she knew she needed backup. Mom called my grandmother back in Louisiana, who was more than happy to come to Memphis to assist with the caregiving but more importantly with the cooking. Whew, did I ever eat? How many skinny teenagers can eat a 12-piece chicken meal with 6 biscuits in one sitting? What about ordering 2-3 full meals when dining at a restaurant? Those feats, though, are not as memorable as the time my friends, family, and I went to Taco Bell for lunch. I ordered a Grande Meal, which consisted of 10 regular tacos, one Burrito Supreme, one Nachos Bell

Grande, and one bonus Mexican Pizza. After eating seven tacos, a friend stated, "Man, you must be getting full." I informed him that it felt like I had not started. Fast food is supposed to be relatively inexpensive, but when you eat as much as 4-6 people by yourself, the costs can add up quickly.

Having eaten everything Taco Bell had to offer, we went to a movie afterwards. On the way out of the theatre, I asked if anyone wanted to stop at Taco Bell on the way home. They busted out laughing and saying, "Yeah right." But I was being dead serious. I felt starved, and that is the insanity that I lived. At the end of the three weeks of being on Dexamethasone, I had gained almost 40 pounds. That's right, 40 pounds in three weeks. Oh my God, my face had ballooned, the size of my rump was stretched to new limits, and I had a gut like a 60-year-old man who drank a case of beer each day. I was unrecognizable to not only others, but my family members and myself (see Figure 1).

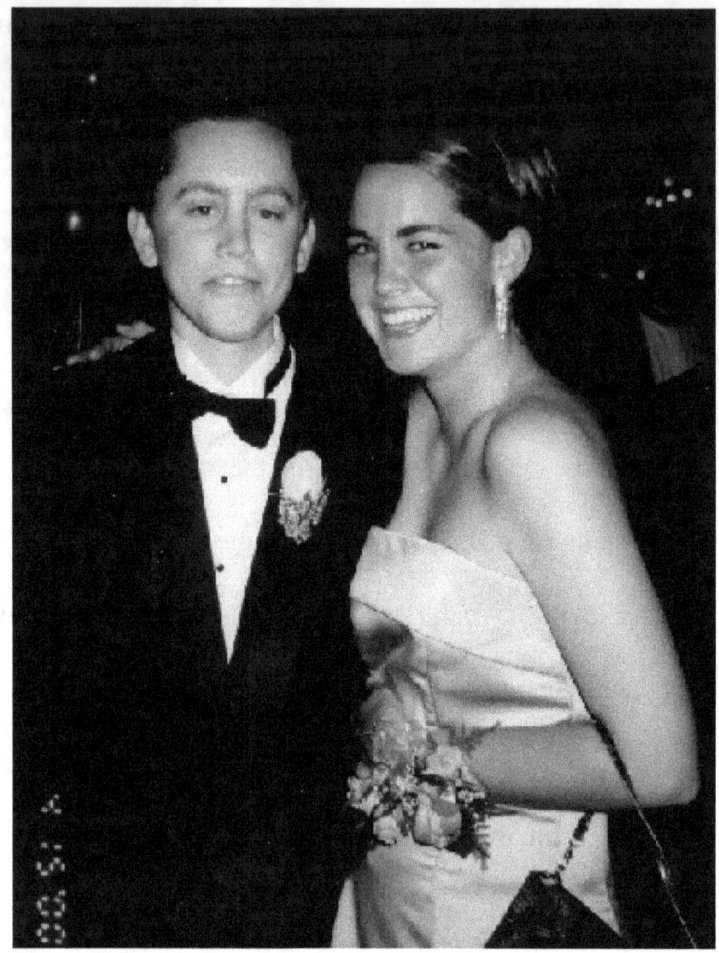
Figure 1. Cushing's syndrome.

Image

Being a young and athletic male, I was rarely concerned about being the 'right' size. Since birth, I was always relatively skinny and never considered weight to be an issue. With the advent of my significant weight gain, I was no longer comfortable within my own skin. I hated the way I looked and was embarrassed for others to see me, because this was not me (see Figure 1). It could not be. It did not even look like me, but instead like a kid who was fat and on his death bed . . . never a good combination.

When the body is exposed to increased levels of Cortisol for a duration of time, side effects include: upper body obesity, rounded face, easily bruised skin that is slow to heal, purplish stretch marks, weakened bones and muscles, fatigue, irritability, anxiety, and depression. Yes, this list sounds like a television advertisement for a sexual dysfunction medication, but they are very real effects from the Dexamethasone that is an essential part of many chemotherapy protocols at St. Jude Children's Research Hospital.

When my mother and others made comments about their figure over the years, I never paid any attention. My thoughts were that those people were strange to be so concerned about how they look in the mirror or to other people. I questioned their self-esteem, since they looked just fine to me. Within a short amount of time, I had that same perspective though. I had become ugly as hell. When I looked in the mirror, I saw a chemo-ridden face, not one of which I was proud. The last day of taking Dexamethasone was one for which I could not wait.

During the fifth week of chemotherapy, I stood in the shower one day just to wash my hair. Clumps of hair began coming off my scalp when I ran my hands through my hair. "Hey Mom, my hair is falling out!" She stood terrified. Mom ran downstairs to the volunteer attendants, Jerry and his wife, asking what to do about my hair. What were they really going to say? In any event, she took it roughly but did gather some information about where I could get my hair cut. I said, "Let's just shave it off tomorrow." She agreed, but it still had an effect on us. I would no longer appear to be the same old Evan. My hair being shaggy in nature gave me a particular appearance that we had grown accustomed to seeing each and every day. We went to the Wal-Mart, as directed by Mr. Jerry at the Ronald McDonald House, where a very kind man shaved it off. As my hair was falling from my head to the floor, the man and my mother began tearing up. On our way out of the salon, Mom suggested that I get an earring to add to my appearance. I smiled but declined the offer to appear any more different than I already did.

The day had come—no more stuffing my face with all the food in sight. Instantly within ceasing to take Dex, my appetite became normalized again. Without maintaining my 8000 calorie diet, I immediately began losing most of the weight that I gained. My maximum weight was 169 lbs, which is not overweight to the average person. That was just over 50 pounds from my sickly weight of 118 lbs at diagnosis. My weight stabilized at around 135 lbs. Not having a gut was a welcoming experience. My parents enjoyed having some money in their wallets too from not spending so much on my constant urges for cuisine.

With a drastic reduction in weight comes other issues, as anyone who has experienced it can attest. Stretch marks! What were these concentrical lines on my butt? My butt looked like the seasonal rings within trees used to determine their age. I did not like the fact that I would always have evidence that I was fat during my life. However, my mother told me some statements that made all the difference. She tried to convince me that they were a normal part of life and that most women who bear a child get them. That was not doing it for me. I was a guy; it was different. I had no excuses for my stretch marks. So she tried a different approach. "Besides, who is going to ever see them besides your mother or your significant other, both of whom will love you regardless of the marks." I could not help but smile. She was right. It did not matter, nor did I really care.

Luckily, that was the only place on my body where the stretch marks remained. I had to keep in mind that there were more important things to worry about than lines on my rear.

There were no limits to which my treatments affected my body. The chemotherapy served to keep me as close to dying as possible. By killing cancerous as well as healthy cells, the chemotherapy targeted rapidly dividing cells. Still, that did not make up for the fact that it was agonizing for nearly every second of every day. There were many things to be joyous about and with which to look forward, but during the ordeal, it was so difficult that it hurts just writing about it today.

Support and determination

If you ever get knocked down, stand up proudly. "Nothing in life can hold you back" was something that my father had told me since I was a young boy. No one could have predicted that those words would provide the basis for continuing to battle with dreaded chemotherapy each week. I relate my struggles to those of Jesus Christ. Now, do not get me wrong. I am no prophet, nor the son of God. I am but a simple person who has experienced some aspects in life, and in those, I have drawn from the teachings of Christianity.

93

With that said, my suffering was not desired by God. However, sometimes we must persist through tough challenges to get to the other side of the equation. My challenges were so much harder than I ever had thought. With a 2 ½ year chemotherapy protocol, it was difficult to feel elation when I knew that there were over two years left of feeling like shit. Although I felt unimaginably miserable most days for two and one-half years, there were always moments of time when life was wonderful. People from numerous states sent me hundreds of post cards—many of whom I did not even know. Through word of mouth, support came in from all over and even above. Individuals from every religion and background informed me that they were keeping me in their thoughts and prayers. I was included on their prayer lists at church. Thousands upon thousands knew of me and I knew only a few of them.

Others offered their condolences through financial assistance in paying for living expenses during my elongated stays in Memphis. My father's colleagues pitched in and hand-delivered two boxes of books, cards, games, toys, and videos to my residence in Memphis. My high school friends even prepared a video that they produced with the assistance of Mr. Fred Aldrich at the television studio at

Baton Rouge Magnet High School. Promoted by my brother, Erich, and my best friend, Joey, a number of people were recruited to give their spirited wishes of goodwill to me from afar. Wow! But to top it off, an envelope was also handed to my father from his associate, Tom Dittman. The envelope contained a bank card of an account with which was established at his employer's credit union. Incredibly, the amount was staggering, totaling over $1800. This was not necessary of these everyday people to give so much consideration to us—an everyday, simple family that was experiencing a tragedy.

Vignette from the day of my attitudinal change

On the days in which high-dose Methotrexate was to be issued, patients were required to have a spinal tap, bone marrow aspirate, and an extended drip of high-dose chemotherapy. Sounds like fun, huh? Having to fast the day of surgery is something all too familiar for chronically ill patients. At St. Jude most teenagers made concerted efforts to eat just before midnight so as not to be terribly hungry the following morning before surgery. However, being 16 and 17 years old during my long-term stays in Memphis meant that most patients were younger than me, since this was a pediatric medical institution. As a result, my procedures and chemotherapy treatments occurred later in the day. The thought process behind this rule was that young children cannot totally understand why they are not allowed to eat and often pitch fits. Indeed, it does seem logical, but it was a burden to bear during those times of heavy steroid use.

Although my procedure was scheduled for 9:00AM, I was not called back until 10:30 for surgery preparation. It became overly ritualistic unfortunately; many Mondays included high-dose chemotherapy during the two induction phases. Telling Mom and Dad goodbye as they left the preparatory room was not overly frightening because of the trust we had in the St. Jude staff. As I was wheeled into the procedure room, I put my game face on—not the one you may be thinking of though. Anything but serious was the manner in which I was composed, as I spoke with the nurses and anesthesiologist about how I was going to fight the drugs they would be issuing.

Versed was always the first medication injected into my bloodstream. It is a short-acting benzodiazepine with a short half-life. Thus, it is perfectly suited for short procedures like the spinal tap and bone marrow aspirate. A feeling of tiredness, haziness, and an accompanied tingling sensation is what I associated with this drug. Yet, I remained fully conscious and able to communicate as normal.

Propofol, on the other hand, was the real deal. Painful going in, Propofol has immediate effects on the body. Its primary use is as a short-acting intravenous sedative agent. When I saw the white stuff in the bottle, I knew my competition had come. This was what I looked forward to each time. Sadistic? Yes. Worthwhile fight? Affirmative. I fought the effects of Propofol in each of our 20-something meetings. Although admittedly I did not stand a chance, it never stopped me from trying to withstand the effects. I always hoped and begged the anesthesiologist to push it slowly, but often he/she did not listen. Those doctors probably thought I was crazy. My method of madness was to begin counting to see how high I could get before the medicine knocked me out. The highest I ever remember counting was about 14; however, the nurses said that I once counted to 27—one of my premier accomplishments in life. In all seriousness though, life is what we make of it. When we are handed these hardships, we make the best of them because that is all we can do. Sedative games like the one mentioned here were just ways that I, as a sick boy, found amusement in the least-amusing time of my life. It is no surprise that even today I find games to be a release from complicated dilemmas of life.

But wait! There is more . . . much more. That was just a description of up to the injection of sedative drugs. While under sedation, doctors regularly completed two tasks: injecting intrethecal Methotrexate via a spinal tap, and conducting a bone marrow aspiration. The spinal tap was unique because of the process of introducing chemotherapy to the region. Nurse practitioners typically completed this relatively straight-forward procedure. They inserted a needle into the lower lumbar region between two vertebrate, withdrew 5ccs of spinal fluid, and injected 5ccs of Methotrexate into the cerebrospinal fluid to prevent lymphomas/leukemias from entering around the spine and brain. Simple enough . . . on paper anyway.

I learned very quickly that there were methods to minimize the discomfort I experienced associated with these procedures. After getting constant, terrible headaches that affected every facet of life, I learned a couple secrets of the trade. Here is a list of three helpful notions to remember when receiving a lumbar puncture:

1. Request that a Sprout needle be used during the procedure. Sprout needles are smaller and typically used for pediatric patients. Some facilities do not carry them; although, the use of Sprout needles has grown since the 1999-2001 era.

2. After the procedure is completed, continue lying down for duration up to four hours. Many nurses will not like that you are occupying their bed space for this length of time, so insist that it is necessary because you have a history of spinal headaches and this has helped you in the past.

3. Keep a urine container nearby. Whatever you do, do not get up when you feel the urge to urinate. Because of the high amount of fluid pumped into you afterwards, this need to urinate will arise soon after waking from the anesthesia.

The bone marrow aspirate (BMA) is completed on the back portion of the hipbone. Although there are different positions that a patient can be placed, I always lied on my side with my knees close to my chest (curled up), also known as the lateral decubitus position.

This also had to do with me getting intrathethical Methotrexate into my spinal column. Thirty minutes prior to the procedure, a nurse cleaned the area and applied some local analgesic cream to numb the area. Then, a needle was inserted through the skin, into the bony cortex, and finally into the marrow cavity. In a twisting fashion, a syringe is used to aspirate the liquid bone marrow out of the bone.

This procedure rarely has any complications and very few side effects are associated with it, other than the patient being sore in the localized region for about two-three days. The sample of bone marrow is pathologically analyzed for hematopoiesis, or the formation of blood cellular components including platelets, red blood cells, and white blood cells.

The day was just getting started. Following the procedure, I still had a high-dose of Methotrexate (MTX) to receive intravenously. Remember, I was lying flat without lifting up my head because I did not want to risk getting a spinal headache. Why? Because once I had a headache for a month and did not leave my bed for four weeks, except to use the bathroom. Now that is agony. I was not about to experience that ever again and I was up for doing whatever was necessary to avoid spinal headaches at any cost.

The high dosages of MTX were always brutal on my body. As an antimetaboite, its use in high doses causes toxic effects to rapidly dividing cells of bone marrow and gastrointestinal mucosa; thus, a rescue drug, Leucovorin, also known as a folic acid, is often used to prevent myelosuppression (bone marrow suppression) or mucositis (the inflammation and ulceration of the mucous membranes lining the digestive tract). This medication has to be taken beginning 24 hours after receiving a high dose of MTX.

As a result of its functionality, Methotrexate is a mainstay in many chemotherapy regimens for various types of cancer. Of course, like any other chemotherapy I received, it made me nauseous to the point of wanting to reach for a gun. There were also a host of side effects associated with this form of chemotherapy like anemia, neutropenia, increased risks of bruising, vomiting, dermatitis, and diarrhea.

There was one more drug with which I detested more than any other. So much so that I did not even take it each time because of the God-forbidden way it made me feel every second of the day. On weeks in which I received the Methotrexate, I also received 6-Mercaptopurine, also known as 6-MP. The drugs work in specific ways to target specific cellular processes and in combination, have been proven to be very effective in killing cancerous cells. This drug was especially hard for me because it was to be taken by mouth (PO), which meant twice a day I had to choose to swallow immediate and prolonged nausea in the form of a pill. Just thinking about it makes my body tremble seven years after having last taken the medication.

On one day in particular during induction, something would be different. While being connected to the bag of MTX, I became courageous. Watching the nurse connect a liter of yellow-colored death in a bag to my IV pole was never fun. But instead of frowning and crying, I smiled the whole time I received the chemotherapy (see Figure 2). Even as I vomited and dry-heaved the remainder of the day, nothing could bring a frown to my face. I had come to the realization and purpose of my sickness—to bring people together. No longer would chemotherapy faze me because I realized that I was stronger than any drug or cancer for that matter. And I had something larger to accomplish in life. I used the cancer to begin the process of unifying my broken family, other families, and circles of friends. Being on the verge of death each day brought my family

closer together.

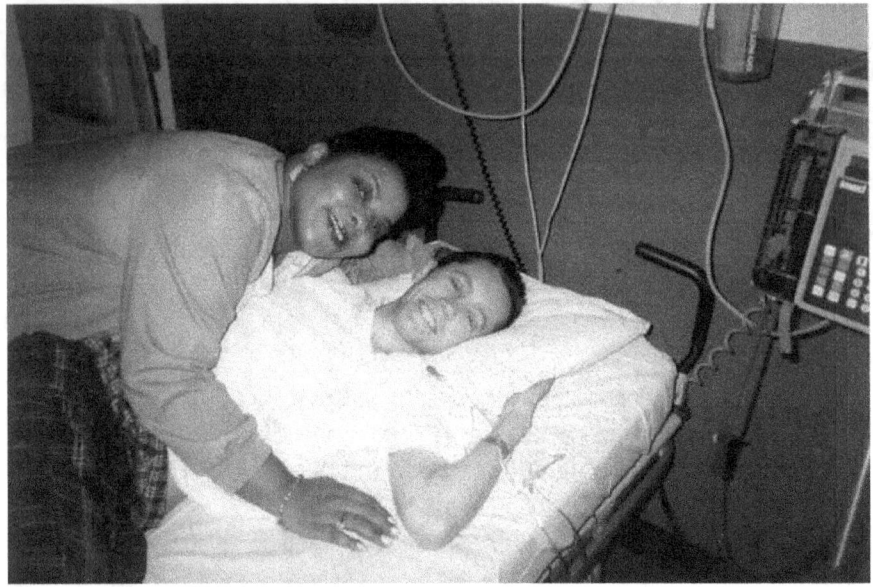

Figure 2. Unflappable smile.

Chapter 6:

A Week in My Shoes

The most common and also most challenging question to

answer is how does chemotherapy make you feel? At a recent

collegiate speaking engagement, I answered the young woman's

question with: "Imagine acid is being fed into your bloodstream."

Although that depiction is partially true, I was not satisfied that I failed to get the feelings associated with cancer and chemotherapy across to one who has never experienced it firsthand. I contemplated about how else I could explain something that is so grueling that words do not do justice for the pain felt by the patient. I could always experience it all again if I so desired, as I still had some remaining 6MP in pill form to be taken by mouth. Nah, the entire reason I still had those pills was that I did not always take them when I was supposed to during the regiment. That was a possibility that was quickly thrown off the list. Shooting a video might allow people to see just how devastating the effects of chemotherapy are as it ravages the body, but people are easily turned off by graphic visual depictions that merely depress the viewer. The only method in which I could transfer these feelings was using the approach of textual depiction through human emotion and experience. Through providing a sample week during my induction phase in Memphis, the reader can gain some clarity about how it feels to undergo regimens of chemotherapy.

Location: St. Jude Children's Research Hospital, Memphis, TN

Residence at the Ronald McDonald House

June 28, 1999

104

Monday

Waking up to my mother saying, "Get ready to go to the hospital . . . we have 20 minutes until we have to leave." It felt like sirens were going off in my head. I became anxious because the previous week I received a high-dose of chemotherapy that almost killed me. This week, however, would be my first of the 10 scheduled weeks of induction therapy. It was designed to nuke the cancerous cells in my body so that I would be in remission in a matter of weeks. I prayed that it would not be like last week.

I had a 7:30AM lab appointment where they would check my counts to measure the effect chemo has had on my body's blood and organ function. I waited approximately 20 minutes before being called to the back. My blood pressure was measured before I was asked to remove my shoes so their weight could be measured. This would prevent me from having to remove my shoes when being weighed each day. I thought that it was an ingenious approach. Another nurse came into the room. She wore a name tag that said 'Line Nurse' below her name. Apparently, she was brought in to prepare an intravenous (IV) line. She said that the most common place was the back of the hand. That did not stop it from hurting though. It felt weird having an IV taped to my hand. When she finished, the other nurse showed me some numbing cream that she suggested she apply to my lower back. Since I would be receiving intrathecal (IT) Methotrexate, which involved a doctor withdrawing spinal fluid and replacing it with chemotherapy, the numbing cream was supposed to reduce the soreness at the injection site. Needless to say, I was more concerned with the procedure and less concerned about temporary soreness. When the nurse finished applying the cream, I was sent back to the waiting room prior to my appointment upstairs in the procedure room.

Again, my name was called to return to A Clinic, where Gwyn walked my mother and me to the elevator. We took the elevator to the third floor, where my mom waited while I was sent back to the procedure room. In a matter of minutes, I was positioned in a hospital gown with my IV connected to fluids. Nurses spoke to me, asking me redundant questions that I had already been asked like, "When is the last time you have eaten/drunk anything?" Then the anesthesiologist walked in the futuristic-looking room that was lit with many lights, which also seemed to be getting colder by the minute. Just wearing a gown and medical socks did not keep me warm enough in the room.

He said hello and informed me that I would be receiving two drugs: Versed and Propofol. The first would calm me down, and the second would knock me out almost immediately. "Sounds good to me," I retorted. The last thing I wanted was to be awake for the procedure, which is how many adults received the same procedure. Not at St. Jude though and I was relieved for that. A nurse prepared my IV with an alcohol packet and then injected some saline to insure the line was clear. Then, the anesthesiologist administered the Versed slowly. About 30 seconds to a minute later, I began feeling a tingling sensation throughout my body. I was not about to fall asleep, but it did make me sleepy-eyed and calm. Meanwhile, several other assistants came in the room, readying themselves for the procedure. The anesthesiologist gave the order, and the Propofol was pushed into my IV. I figured that it could not have as much effect on my body as he had stated earlier. Still, I followed the doctor's orders of taking a couple of deep breaths. The solution felt extremely cold going into my veins, resembling a burning sensation. My next memory was awakening in the recovery room from a blood pressure cuff making noise, as it automatically measured my pressure every five minutes. "How are you feeling?," a nurse asked. "Like I just woke up from a procedure," I sarcastically replied. "Not too bad though." She asked me what I would like to drink, since I had to take a few sips of a beverage before I could leave the recovery room. I proposed that a Sprite would be nice, so she retrieved the beverage. When she returned, my mother followed her into the room. "Hey Ev," she said in a nurturing tone. It hurt her to see me lying in bed recovering from a procedure. She assisted me by holding the cup next to my mouth, just as she had done in my early childhood years. I didn't mind the help because I still had an IV in one of my hands, and since I was still lying on one of my sides from having the procedure between two of my lower vertebrae.

Once I passed their tests of maintaining a stable blood pressure and could keep liquids down, they wheeled me down to the first floor and into the lobby. They said that I could continue to use the wheelchair for as long as I needed. For any normal hospitalization, this would have been the end of the day but not here. That was just the commencement to a full-fledged battery of torture. That is why I thought it was a good idea not to exert undue energy in walking through the hospital to the lunch room. Feeling something squeamish from the sedation, I was hesitant to eat but my hunger won out. Mom wheeled me to the lunchroom so that I could eat something light before the afternoon appointments and chemotherapy.

It was just after 1:00PM by this time, and the regular lunch line had already closed. The only options for cuisine were hamburgers, fries, chicken wings, and desserts. It was sure time to eat, but my stomach was sending my brain mixed signals. Although my hunger was challenged by my feelings of nausea, chicken wings, corn, and a roll were my choices for lunch with some Sprite to wash it down. Mom brought our trays to the counter, where we redeemed our lunch vouchers, which amazingly covered the entire cost of the meal for both my mother and me. While we were eating, I could tell it was hard for mom to eat much of her food, as she watched me slowly taking bites here and there. She was very uncomfortable seeing me in a condition other than an athletic, extraverted teenager. Pushing food around my plate and not talking much was a stark contrast to my ordinary self. She did drink her Diet Coke, which I would not have touched with a 10-foot pole. Having once tasted it by accident, the after taste was in no way worth the potential hydration. I ate most of the chicken, two spoons of the corn, and one bite of the roll. It was not very tasty. We had to get going anyhow, because it was nearing 2:00PM—my appointment time at the medicine room. We proceeded back to the waiting area until we were finally called into the medicine room at 2:45. I suppose that they were behind, and so I waited and waited and waited. It was interesting to wait for something that would likely cause pain on my body because I would have just as well taken a hiatus to the Rocky Mountains. In the past, I was only accustomed to waiting outside of electronic stores on Black Friday for potential deals. That was the extent to which I waited. Ultimately, one of the nurses greeted me at the door and I followed her inside.

Mom wheeled my chair into this huge room with dozens of beds lined up in four rows, resembling a military barracks. Curtains were drawn between each of the beds, but privacy seemed like it would be at a minimum. Still, I was more concerned with what lied ahead in regard to the chemotherapy regiment. Just the week before was my first experience with chemotherapy. The high-dose of Methotrexate served as a knockout punch, and I was dreadful of

110

what this week's regiment would hold. I proceeded to the side of the room to urinate before being hydrated even more before the issuing of the chemotherapy. Walking towards my mother, I took off my shoes and sat on the bed. Propping myself in the bed, throwing the sheets over half my body, and trying desperately to find some comfort followed. Once again, I was hooked up to more fluids. This seemed redundant but again, I followed the rules of their game. Hanging the fluids on the IV pole and programming the machine to administer 100cc/hr, the nurse said that she would be back in a little while once the fluids had a chance to get going. Meanwhile, she would call the pharmacist to acquire my chemotherapy. Really? My very own chemotherapy. Just for me? How sweet . . . you shouldn't go out of your way to get it? Really, you don't have to. Those were my thoughts; none of which were voiced. After my programmatic machine began beeping randomly due to air in the line, I was prepped to receive the chemo about 30 minutes from my arrival in the medicine room (3:15PM). Not too bad in terms of waiting time. But less waiting time also equated with chemotherapy coming sooner. No matter what happened, the outcomes were not enjoyable.

Although it was just 30 minutes, time was in no way flying by because I was uncomfortable, anxious, and not quite feeling right from the anesthesia earlier in the morning. Thank God I had my mother by my side. Mom kept asking me questions like, "What can I do?" I did not know the answer. Was there something that she could have done for me to feel less nauseous, worried, and scared?

Cindy, the nurse, returned with my chemotherapy. She was always smiling and friendly, while my demeanor was unlike hers. Grumpy and quiet, I did not want to chit chat. "Let's do it and get it over with," I uttered. She complied, hung the Vincristine and Daunomyacine on the pole, started the drips, and pulled the curtain behind her on her way out. I took a deep breath, because I knew the worst was soon to come. A few minutes into the ordeal, I looked to my arm, seeing the chemotherapy feeding through the line, into the needle, and into my veins. It made me sick just looking at it. My body felt different too. All over. Just a yucky feeling from which I could not run away. And then, the taste in my throat. The more I swallowed, the worse it became. I curled up in the fetal position, crying on the inside. There were hours to go; this was just the beginning.

My feelings of nausea built, but they were different than the normal bouts of nausea one might feel. Typically, I could vomit and the nausea would subside. Not with chemo though. Everything was exacerbated, from the nausea to the pain to the loneliness to the mood swings to the depression. These ideas were fixated within my mind each and every day. Wishing you were dead is not advisable, but it went with the territory. Nothing imaginable was or is as bad as undergoing chemotherapy. Broken bones, car accidents, burns, sicknesses, nothing. In fact they don't even come close to the savagery with which one's body is put through.

I still could not vomit though, so there was nothing to do but close my eyes and dream. Dream of a better place, but how? My symptoms intensified constantly so that now was worse than several minutes ago, and several minutes from now will be even worse. Self-induced vomiting was the only thing that my mother and I could come up with. So after trying to vomit on my own, I started sticking my finger down my throat so as to cause myself to gag, hoping this would stimulate regurgitation. It didn't work at first, but with some effort, I finally vomited in the bucket that my mother fetched for me minutes before. Great, now I had vomit remnants in my nose, throat,

113

and on my sheets. The unpleasant experience lingered with me for another 15 minutes until I could get situated again. The toll that it took on me was apparent. My sides hurt, heart was beating fast, and I was sweating. All the while, the IV was still pumping more chemo into my bloodstream. The nausea subsided slightly at best, but I could not fall asleep or anything because my body was so worked up by that point. This spout of vomiting occurred once again while I was in the medicine room that day. Tasting vomit became too familiar for me, and mixed with the funky taste that the chemo left me with, I must have had spectacular breath that day.

Hours later, the drip finished so I sat up and decided to jolt for the bathroom. I had to urinate so badly after holding it in forever due to intravenous fluids being given all the while to clean out the poisonous chemo from my body. Just getting out of the bed was a draining experience. I did not think that much about it though because I was so sick of lying in that bed all afternoon. Urinating was quite memorable because of the smell. The pungent odor was not pleasant and I supposed that it indicated a high level of toxicity that my body contained from the intravenous chemotherapy just issued. Finally, I was unhooked from the machine, my IV was removed, and I was free to leave the hospital . . . for the day.

My mother decided that it would be a wise decision to return to the lunchroom because neither one of us felt like preparing anything to eat back at the Ronald McDonald House. Mom wheeled me through the hospital to the lunchroom, while I thought about something I would be interested in eating for dinner. I honestly did not feel like eating. The fear of upchucking any food was not worth the risk. Nevertheless, I saw the chicken drummies behind the counter and had to give them a try. They looked so tasty. Besides, they were my favorite lunchtime selection, and I did not want to risk my appetite on the other choice—meatloaf. I also ordered green beans. With the meal, I took my second dose of Prednisone (another steroid), which I took by mouth with each meal of the day as part of my weekly regimen of pharmaceutical drugs.

Beginning to eat, the chicken tasted yummy. Then again, anything was better than the taste that was already in my mouth. Several minutes later, though, the effects of the chemotherapy worsened. I tried desperately to delay puking so as to get some nourishment from the food but it did not work. I didn't even have time to run to the bathroom, so I was forced to vomit in the small plastic container that my mother happened to have in her purse. Suddenly, I ripped into full vomit lunging forward barely securing the plastic container, but my vomit was not controlled enough to entirely land in the container, so some of it went on the lunch room table. I was saddened that I threw up. Someone would have to clean it up, and in addition, I made a big scene while others were trying to eat their dinner. No one wanted to see someone puking while they ate their soup and salad.

As if something were brewing deep in my bellows, this feeling came from my core. My lower back began hurting as well as other joints too. It was as if my gag reflex was in constant perturbation. Dry heaving for 15 minutes ensued before getting wheeled to the front doors of the building. I should have stuck with my initial inkling of not eating that night. Mom and I took the shuttle to the Ronald McDonald House. I walked into the building passing some children outside playing together, went into the building, straight to the elevator, up to the second floor, into my room to lie down on the bed, got under the sheets, curled up in a ball, and prayed that my misery would go away. "God, please, please just make me feel normal again. I beg you to help me to get through this with as little agony as possible. I know that it is almost inevitable, but give me the strength that is necessary to make it through this week. I love you."

We turned on the fans, air purifiers, and the air conditioning to drown out all the noises from the facility. Any visual or auditory engagement was overstimulation of the senses. My body needed solitude, peace, tranquility, and silence. I slept for about two hours and by the time I woke up, it was around 8:00PM. Mom asked if I was up to eating something. Eventually, I heeded her advice and said that I would like some grits. Hopefully, my stomach would tolerate the simple meal. Still trying to calm down, I remained curled up in bed as she brought the food to my side. Wanting it to be tomorrow, I sat up while I ate some grits for dinner. The grits tasted mediocre, but it was likely because of the chemo they tasted that way. I began to calm down as I finished my meal. This temporary sensation was interrupted quickly though as my vomiting episodes returned 45 minutes later. Taking several trips to the bathroom to hang my head over the toilet, I gave up. Nothing would come out. It always felt like puking was inevitable, but still, the nausea persisted. I contemplated

117

sleeping next to the toilet that night but finally returned to bed, lied

back down, asked my mom for the room to be completely dark, and

fell asleep once my body could not tolerate another second of the

day. I was in a state of complete exhaustion. All I could do was pray

and cry myself to sleep.

Tuesday

Waking up at 7:30AM was not for me. There was no way I

would ordinarily awaken this early in the summertime, but I had no

choice because of some appointments at the hospital. The recurrent

dire need to urinate from being hydrated via intravenous fluids was

blatantly apparent and was the overbearing reason that I quickly

arose from my slumber. As I walked to the restroom located in the

room, it was very different from any other morning. Each step felt

like I had been standing for 24 hours straight . . . foot pain, leg pain,

shoulder soreness, back aches, and the back of my hand felt bruised

from the IV yesterday.

I sat hunched over on the toilet because it took too much

energy to sit up straight. The lights were off, leaving a crack between

the door and the bedroom so as not to turn on the light, because lights were incredibly straining on my eyes. I always kept the curtains drawn shut to keep the room shaded too.

As I urinated, the urge to vomit came over me. In mid-stream it was impossible to get off the toilet and prepare oneself for an episode of vomiting, so I pushed my urine out as fast as possible. Then, I tried but could not force my body to heave, so the feelings of nausea persisted. Seconds later, looking at myself in the mirror served as a visual reminder that this newfound life was very real. It was no dream or nightmare for that matter; I was undergoing chemotherapy. Seeing my fatigued face and hair in disarray, I turned to the side just before ripping off my bandage from my lower back area from the site of the IT. Checking my body was natural to me. So after removing the bandages, I lightly touched near that area, evaluating the level of soreness/pain. The location of the intrusion between vertebrae was associated with a sharp pain. Although this may seem obvious, it was still very new to me. I told mom, "I wish they made cushion bandages, because it would help buffer the trauma throughout the day."

I put on some shorts and a t-shirt, brushed my teeth, ran a brush through my hair and realized that it was only 8:00AM. I still had 30 minutes before we had to leave. The shuttle service came downstairs every 30 minutes, so as long as I was downstairs before 8:30AM, we were in business. With mom's approval, I napped a bit longer, as the bed provided a place of solace for which I desperately sought. What seemed like 20 seconds later, but in actuality was 20 minutes, my mother woke me to walk downstairs and prepare myself for what the day entailed. Other families were also waiting for the shuttle; luckily there was still room to fit in the 10-person van.

Arriving once again at the hospital, which was right on the other side of the interstate from the Ronald McDonald House, I checked in, attained my wrist bracelet, and headed to the lab for my daily blood work. I had a 9:00AM lab appointment and a 10:30AM appointment to have intramuscular (IM) Asparaginase shot administered in the medicine room. Just thinking about that room made me quiver. It was just yesterday that I received a chemotherapy drip over several hours there. I was still nauseous from it, and they were going to compile my nausea with more cell-destroying substances. That didn't seem right to me, but again, I put my utmost confidence in the doctors and their research-based experimental programs and chemotherapy regiments. While waiting for the lab appointment, I sat watching other patients and their families. Their appearances varied from normal to weak and discolored faces. Some children looked to be on their last days of life.

The waiting room was filled with games and supplies as well as volunteers who gave the patients and their siblings the best experience possible while at the hospital. The major quagmire was that no matter what games were provided to act as distractions from the pain that these patients were feeling; it seemed like a hopeless endeavor in trying to relieve their pain. Clearly, many of the young patients loved painting, socializing with the other children, and constructing art projects, but it was clear that those children were in a different world than the cancer-free individuals beside them. Seeing children as young as 6 weeks old to the age of 17 that day gave me a clearer understanding about how cancer can exist in anyone and without wonderful facilities to diagnose and treat these diseases, these beautiful people's lives would be cut short. I began to feel a bond with other cancer patients there in that we endured undue amounts of grief to live another day of pain in hopes of seeing the other side of life—back to our days of being carefree.

Finally hearing my name called on the hospital intercom system, I walked back into A Clinic for my medical evaluation that preceded any issuance of chemotherapy. I met with Gwyn, my primary nurse, and she gave me a printout of my blood count information and explained that the levels were all within normal range. I grabbed the paper from Gwyn, seeing a list of 30 or so indicators and their numerical descriptors. Almost all of the information was incomprehensible to my untrained eye. Shortly later, Dr. Sandlund entered the room wearing a smile on his face. He said that he was excited to see me again; his sincerity showed too. He inquired as to how I was feeling as he began to do his physical examination, which included the following routine: look in my ears, eyes, feel neck for lymph nodes, listen to carotid artery, look in mouth, listen to stomach by palpating and percussing stomach /percuss back to listen to lungs in back and front, listen to heart, lie me down, check pulse in arms and feet, and check testicles for lumps. He continued to check for muscle strength/reflexes in cranial nerves, pupil area, extraocular movements, smiling, eyelid closing, shoulder shrug, stick out tongue, biceps, triceps, knee up/down, leg ups, feet push/pulls.

Answering his question about how I was feeling proved to be as difficult as writing this memoir. I had no background experience in dealing with elongated periods of nausea so describing how I felt proved to be tricky. This is what I wish I would have stated: the rubber band tourniquet, alcohol prep, needle, and my arm—a scene that flashed over and over again in my mind. Too many times and still the nurses' words were never heard. It was the visual that was surreal—the instruments, the atmosphere of others in pain, the smell of take-out lunches, and the constant drone of children yelling. These events added to my sensory perceptions being overloaded. Making my veins rise to the surface of my pale skin, my efforts allowed the needle to be pushed into my vein. Deeper, the feelings of hurt increased, but the pain reminded me that I could still feel . . . that is until the chemo comes later. I thought, "Now I see how drug users feel—they use blockers to null the pain they associate with life." I wished there were counteractive agents that provided relief from the chemotherapy, but in my experiences, there was no match for the poisonous substances associated with the medications in my regimen. It was the calm before the storm, the silence before the attack. The environment was eerie as I watched nurses, patients, and family members. Nurses wheeled out trays of materials and brought out bags of liquid to hang and whenever they included chemotherapy, their faces said it all. Sometimes they would even tell you flat out, "I'm sorry I have to do this." Tell me about it . . . so was I. Bags were hung, IV machines tuned to drip at specific amounts per hour, and then it began. Pure, unadulterated, cringe-filled destruction ensued.

Mom, dad, or my brother, whoever happened to be in the room, observed as I tried to watch television to serve as a distraction. Some children asked for sheets to be thrown over the liquid bags of chemotherapy because they associated the red bag or the orange bag with the recurrent symptoms and feelings that followed. It didn't matter to me. I was there to receive the death-like substances, although I must admit that I also associated bearing degrees of nausea with certain drugs as would anyone.

It starts to drip at a steady rate and I watch. I look at my IV, following it from the bag to the machine, still following it for another five feet or so until where it is connected in my arm. I watch as it goes into my body, knowing it is killing cells of all kinds, disrupting protein synthesis, and in all kinds of other ways to interrupt cell division. Minutes into this administering of chemo, I start to feel awful inside. It seemed that my intestinal tract was the primary area with which chemo was felt, however, it was actually the posterema part of the brain sending signals to that area. Still, the queasiness was worsening by the minute, but the bag remained near full. Unlike a child who touches a hot stove and learns to remove his hand, I could not go anywhere. There was no escape from its havoc. Nowhere to run or hide. And no one to bring any relief. Comfort was nonexistent, merely a façade fading away. With each additional minute of the substances filtering into my bloodstream came upchucking, drained energy levels, and muscle weakness.

I lie there and try to run my hands through my hair but remember one is still connected to a machine. I cry. What the hell is this? This is what life is. Give me a break. The tears run down my face even at this moment as I write. I place the palms of my hands over my eyes blocking out the outside world. The tears cover my face. I try to hold on to the life I once had, but it doesn't exist anymore. I utter a scream for salvation but nothing comes out but mumbled sounds of strain. Spitting out tears and blowing my nose for durations of time solves no problems but it provides me with a

125

reminder that I have a tremendous spirit that is nearing ruin. This much pain served as an appetizer to the next two plus years, and it alone was next to intolerable, but it served as a reminder that 99% of the time when not undergoing chemotherapy, life is free of hurt and pain. Perhaps one day I could just be a regular guy again.

I feel as though my gag reflex is in constant perturbation. My mouth stays open and over a bucket because at any time Mount St. Helens could erupt. Nauseous feelings circulate through the body like the blood in its circulatory system, providing life to both its organs and the nerve endings that make me feel like I am dying. My insides want to be free of my internal chambers so they jolt in unison with my incredibly powerful spats of heaving. My vomiting resembles the force of someone receiving the Heimlich maneuver over and over again until finally well beyond the time when there is nothing left in my stomach to churn, my body gives in to the demons and says enough. Sweating, beaten, and winded, the body stops fighting. Feeling taken advantage of, you have nothing left to give the world for the chemotherapy has raped you of your humility and innocence.

Outsiders wonder why some cancer patients have bad attitudes, negative demeanors, and tainted views on life. This is why! It is not their wish; it is that their souls have been stripped from their being. Like those who have the plague, cancer patients feel like outcasts of society. They look different, undergo sickness, and simply seek out love and affection. Their feelings are of concern to outsiders, as long as they stay out of sight and out of mind. Jaded as one can be, the mindset that life sucks is evident to many. But it is that these people have not seen the other side again that they once experienced. They are incapable of knowing how beautiful life can be until the chemo is over, just as someone who has never experienced it firsthand cannot fathom what having cancer entails. Those foreign feelings do not allow connections and relationships to flourish. Until you see from their perspective, you will never know so give them the benefit of the doubt and go the extra mile with kindness, compassion, and concern.

As Dr. Sandlund continued with his workup, everything seemed to check out nicely except my reflexes. They were limited in the knee area, but with some diligence, he was able to make one of the two twitch. Sandlund and I made small talk before he discussed the Asparaginase shot that I would be administered. Informing me that generally patients did not have any issues like nausea associated with it, I was pleasantly surprised. So all chemotherapy did not have the same side effects? This was exciting news and I had a glimmer of hope for the day! I still felt the effects from the previous day but just knowing that it would not be compounded from today was reassuring. This particular shot did have potential side effects like hypotension and/or respiratory complications. Whatever . . . I never paid any attention to side effects for any of the medications I had taken growing up, because there were always 10 times the side effects as the use of the drugs. Those were also in rare cases that the side effects occurred. Not a concern for me, although I had never received a shot in my leg. It seemed slightly awkward, but I was ok with it, understanding the idea of intramuscular shots.

We sat in the waiting room for another hour—sitting, watching, and closing my eyes, as I heard babies crying and children playing. Again, those unforgettable words, "Evan Ortlieb, please come to the medicine room." I stood up like I had won the lottery, and in one way, I had. I did not have to remain waiting and waiting any longer. I sat in one of the seats in the room that was tilted in just

a position so as to lounge, which fit my personality just fine.
Tapping my hands on the arm rests like drums seemed to be my way
of dealing with my anxiety that day. This would be my first time
receiving the Asparaginase shot. The nurse, Patty, said that it would
be given in the quadriceps area of my right leg. She took my blood
pressure and then left to pick up the medication from the pharmacy. I
spoke with my mom about the situation. "Mah, what do you think?"
"Not really sure," she said. "It can't be as bad as the large drips that
you received yesterday." I agreed. Her words seemed to settle my
nerves until the nurse back. She walked towards me, pushing the
wheeled tray. The tray only contained two items: an alcohol prep and
the pre-filled syringe containing Asparaginase. She told me that the
Asparaginase prevented the cancer cells from growing, which was
what I figured since it was a form of chemotherapy. It was
nevertheless reassuring before being stuck that it was not Botox for
cosmetic purposes. "This is going to burn," she said. I thought about
how in the world the needle could burn me, and then I realized to
what she was referring. She stuck the needle in my leg and began
pushing the liquid inside the muscle. "Yikes!" The burning sensation
came from the liquid substance protruding into my muscle. It felt

about 10 times worse than a cortisone shot—the only other time I can remember substances being pushed into my muscles. Not only did it burn, but the amount of liquid was seemingly much more than I thought could possibly be pushed into the area. "God, hurry up," I thought. "When will she ever finish?" Almost jumping out of my seat, I had to focus so diligently not to leap out of the chair. She eventually finished and said, "See, not that bad, huh?" I politely disagreed.

I held some gauze over the area while the nurse prepared a bandage. She placed it on and informed me that I had to stay in the room for 30 minutes. "Lucky me," I thought. I didn't really feel like walking anywhere to be honest. My leg was still incredibly sore in the area in which the Asparaginase was administered. Mom and I looked at one another, and I just shook my head. She still had the look of "Ouch, that has to hurt" on her face from several minutes ago. I sat back trying to relax and eventually I could deal with the pain, because it was just that—pain. Nausea was not accompanied with it, and I hoped the onset would not occur either. Watching television allowed the 30 minutes to pass slightly faster than just sitting there, even though I paid no attention to what I was watching.

Turning channels using a wired remote did little but remind me I was in a hospital facility, so I just put it down and left it alone.

The nurse returned after I sent mom for her. We were hungry for lunch so we were sure to watch the time since the shot. Just as we were departing, Patty said that I had to return one hour from then for a final check. "OK," I said. Mom and I pushed the doors open simultaneously. On the other side of the door, we began walking to the cafeteria discussing whether or not we would return to the medicine room afterwards. We were content with doing a self-check and heading out, but we would ultimately decide at the end of lunch.

Lunch was standard—the cafeteria was busy, full of families, practitioners, and researchers eating while still maintaining discussions about work. The life of the physicians seemed to revolve around their highly talented craft and as a patient, I was truly thankful for their dedication. That level of passion is both a strength and the eventual undoing of hard workers. Mom ate a salad she prepared from the fixings available; apparently, it was tasty because she finished it all. I, on the other hand, had a full meal of a hamburger, seasoned fries, chips, Sprite, and a fudgesicle. Mom and I agreed that I should eat the fudgesicle first; after all, how many

131

times do you get to eat a free fudgesicle that was looking tastier by the second. I could have used the excuse that my leg was still throbbing from the Asparaginase shot, but it was never necessary with mom.

Leaving the cafeteria, I decided that it was not the proper time to break the rules for which I signed my name to just two weeks before, so we headed back to the medicine room. Patty looked at my leg. It showed no signs of a chemical reaction so we were free to leave at last. Should we check out the city? Tour the area? Nah, let's hit the sack back at the Ronald McDonald House. Getting out of the hospital was first on our list though so we left the medicine room, went to the front of the hospital doors, and waited on the shuttle pickup service. As I approached the van, it was filling up rapidly and luckily, mom and I got on the van as I had the privilege of riding in the front passenger seat. The driver said I had to be the navigator and I gladly agreed as long as I could get in the van; meanwhile, both of us knew that I knew nothing of the city or how to travel anywhere. I smiled.

We exited the van. I shut the doors and walked through the entrance of the Ronald McDonald House, passing some older family

132

members hanging out on the front benches while their children and grandchildren played nearby. I walked in and headed directly upstairs. I didn't want to socialize, snack, secure something to drink, or watch television. I just wanted to hide under my sheets and go to sleep. Was I tired? Not really, but the bed was my place of relief. I could go there and always feel better than standing around, sitting up, or walking somewhere. The bed and its pillows were my best friends that day—one pillow for my head, one between my legs, and the last between my arms. Snuggling myself to nap was thoroughly enjoyable and a delightful getaway from the day-to-day hospital experiences. Plus I did not have anything connected to me—no needles, lines, or bandages.

Coming in and out of consciousness, I finally sat up, looking to the right where my mom's bed was. She was content reading a book in a room with no light, except for the book light that hung from the top of the page. Mom kept her Stephen King and John Grisham books close by to pass the time. I later learned that she had difficulties being away from home. In fact she hated being there and living at the Ronald McDonald House. Whenever she returned to Baton Rouge though, she remained in an uneasy state. Mom didn't feel normal back in Baton Rouge either, desiring to get back to Memphis as soon as possible. The push and pull of having part of an immediate family in Memphis, Tennessee, while having the others in Baton Rouge, Louisiana was taking its toll on my mother. By the time we finally returned to Baton Rouge for good, mom still felt awkward. She realized that people could sympathize with what was going on in our family and with me, but could not empathize at all. How could they though? They knew as much as we did at the beginning of the process. It was sometimes frustrating though when people would give ignorant remarks like "So you guys are done, right?"

The evening came soon enough as I slept most of the afternoon. When I wasn't sleeping, I walked down the hall to shoot a game or two of billiards. There was no one else in the room, but that suited me just fine. It was a distraction and I did not need any competitors to get me worked up. I was competitive by nature. Soon though, I became bored of hitting the pool balls around so I went back to the room to take a shower and relax. I had not taken one that morning and my hair was still in disarray from my going back to bed that morning, not that it bothered me in the least. I was there for other reasons besides glamorous photoshoots.

Having returned to my bedroom at the Ronald McDonald House, I relished being able to lounge without having millions of concerns. I had just one. In the room the thermostat was always kept on freezing cold. I don't think it said that on the dial, but it was maxed out as cold as it could get. It was always chillingly cold for several reasons including my bouts of random sweating and to push my body to sleep for durations at a time without the desire to wake/get up to the extent that whoever was living with me at the time would have to wear jackets and throw blankets on them to keep from becoming ill. I regularly kept the temperature on the lowest setting 65 degrees in the middle of the summer months.

I did not have a television in my room yet, so there was not much to do in the room except sleep. Before going to bed that night, I ate some dinner that mom prepared in the shared kitchen downstairs. While she upheld her motherly duties for which I am eternally grateful, I watched TV downstairs in the shared living space. For a couple of minutes, I sat in the kitchen, speaking with other families. These leisurely activities were extensions of the non-academic tendencies I held in Baton Rouge. However, this time there was valid reasoning behind my choices. I began to realize that it was hard to focus on one thing for very long before becoming tired, as my eyes felt like shutting. The television screen would wear on my strained eyes. Even still, I found ample opportunities to channel surf before and after eating dinner. My perspective then was the same as it is now—watching television is mostly a waste of time, so it was the perfect device for trying to finish 2.5 years as soon as possible.

Wednesday

Waking up, opening my eyes, pulling off the sheets and blanket from covering my body, and sliding out of the bed as I put my feet on the floor were my first memories of the day. Just four seconds later, the nausea was evident too. I was reminded of the treatment from Monday. Great, I wish I were still sleeping because I was dreading going back to the hospital again. When was this going to stop?

Having to wake up early, 7:30AM, did not help out the cause. I was not a morning person to begin with, nor was I excited about the reason I was awake. Prepping again consisted of very little other than brushing my teeth. A look in the mirror was not even necessary anymore, for I knew that my appearance was diminishing. We soon departed the Ronald McDonald House for assessment and triage at the hospital.

Checking in with Ron, one of the patient services' gurus, was pleasant. Each day we conversed and he was so helpful pointing out that not only were we eligible for meal vouchers, but we should also take a snack pack voucher that could be redeemed after lunch hours. Ron handed over my schedule for the day, which I was already holding a similar printout from yesterday when I left the hospital. Nothing was different, but he pointed out that schedules and doctor appointments were subject to change.

Having already checked in at the hospital and picked up my meal cards, I arrived in the waiting area for assessment and triage. This was the hangout during the early mornings since almost every patient had to go through assessment and triage in the mornings. Overcrowding was sometimes a problem especially when some families had sick and well family members playing, running around, and yelling. I cannot say much negatively about their actions because I would be doing the same if I were in their situation. Once my name was called, I split the crowds walking into my clinic for assessment and triage. My blood pressure and blood samples were taken while I discussed my current status. "Excuse me, ma'am. Can I have the needle inserted in my mid-arm, on the opposite side of my elbow?" The IV in my hand from Monday was still bruised and I had much more flesh in my arm than on the back of my hand. She said that blood work was normally drawn from the arm, but that many times nurses place IVs on the hand so they do not get tangled in clothes. When she agreed that my arm would be a suitable placement, I was deeply relieved. One less thing that would hurt was only a small measure of success but it was something that made me feel better. The pain in my hand lingered and I did not want to feel it ever again if possible. Upon finishing with the preliminary evaluation necessary to provide the doctors with pertinent information to know whether I am in suitable condition for today's procedures and/or how my body is reacting to the medications, I was sent back to the lobby. Why couldn't Dr. Sandlund just come see me then? My single-minded focus never considered that he was seeing 10-20 patients or more that morning.

Afterwards, I sat again in the lobby next to A Clinic. It was evident that many of the patients were called before me. Maybe it was just a coincidence. Finally, Gwyn came out and sent us into a room, saying that she could work us in right then. She didn't have to tell me twice, because I was fed up with waiting. Something about sitting around doing nothing in an environment where suffering was evident was anything but how one would want to spend any amount of time. She seated us in a room, asking preliminary questions for Dr. Sandlund's workup like if we needed any medications/prescriptions. "Dr. Sandlund will be in the room shortly," she said, and I looked forward to seeing him. Something about his demeanor and personality could bring a smile to anyone's face, even in times of strife. Sandlund was always dressed in a particular way that I categorize as classy-casual-sophisticated. His hair was not short, but longer and wavy. He wore a full-smile each time he saw his patients because he cared so much about them in every way, not just physical health.

Mom and I were talking about him saying how he probably lived in midtown in some of the larger, more lavish houses. Maybe even in Germantown, but that was slightly farther out of the city than we expected. Cars? Mom guessed he drove an Infiniti, something classy and a bit sporty. I agreed, and soon thereafter Sandlund asked

139

me how things were going. Naturally, mom and I brought up the issue. Mom rehashed our conversation and inquired. His answer was perfectly suitable and representative of his character: "I drive an old Mitsubishi Eclipse. Nothing really fancy. Why?" "Oh, no reason. We just figured that you look nice and dress with style that your car probably matched." He taught me a lesson without even saying anything. The car one drives has no effect on the individual. Instead it is merely a physical mechanical machine that does one single job and that alone. There are greater things in life with which to focus and about which to be concerned.

After he checked me all around, he sent me to the area in which MRIs were taken. These were once-a-week MRI or X-Ray checks to study the size/location of the tumor in my chest. Again, I waited in the area to be scanned before being called to the room that housed the diagnostic equipment. While waiting for my return, mom went to the lunch room for a soft drink and a snack, remembering to pick up my snack pack for that afternoon. When she came back I was still in the room, so she picked up medical supplies from the pharmacy which included Nystatin rinse, Ondansetron, and a pill splitter.

The MRIs were not difficult or painful, so I never had any complaints about having them. It was somewhat awkward though to have a chamber two inches from your face inside a cylindrical machine. The whole time I lied in this machine I thought about how my mother was claustrophobic and would just about die if she were in this place. I smiled, closed my eyes, and listened to the radio station on the earphones that the attendant handed me minutes ago. He even allowed me to pick the radio station. It was a local rock station, which allowed me to sample the rock music that was popular around town. This was enjoyable and if I was indeed going to be staying in the area for an extended amount of time (the rest of the summer), it made sense to learn about the culture and musical niches that pervaded the community.

As much as I enjoyed listening to the music, it was sometimes hard to hear all of the sounds and words easily as a dramatic series of beeps rang out like the beginning of a war. Enh Enh Enhhhh. Do do do do do, Enh Enh Enh. This pattern continued with intermittent parts of silence for which I was glad. Nevertheless, this was my break from the hideous face of chemotherapy. I should not have ever thought about it, because it was making me sick to even contemplate being back in the medicine room once again.

Finishing the MRIs, I changed back into my clothes from the hospital gown and headed to lunch to get something to eat. There was plenty enough time to get a tall cup of Sprite and some red beans and rice with cornbread. The day's special seemed mighty tasty just looking at it, so I had to do the right thing and give it a try. Being a native Louisianian, I was accustomed to foods that were well-seasoned and spicy. We found a place to sit in the large cafeteria room, picked up our utensils, and then remembered that we needed to pray first. Mom said, "Dear Lord, bless this food that we have before us. Please help it nourish our bodies, especially Evan as he struggles with his chemo treatments. Thank you for letting us find this place, St. Jude Hospital, so that Evan may have the best chance for healing. Please watch over the rest of the family, including Monica, back at home. Amen."

While shoveling in the food, I sat staring at the table. There were distractions all around, but with focus, I could tune a portion of them out. The food on the plates was becoming overwhelming to my eyes, as I began remembering how sick I would soon feel. I continued eating some more though because I knew that my dinner could be almost non-existent for I became accustomed to puking most evenings. It was not always easy knowing that my food needed to be eaten but might be upchucked hours later. This unsettling thought coursed through my mind and before long, it was time to leave the lunch room. My own thoughts and inner workings had distracted me so much that I had no recollection of what mom and I had discussed during the meal.

Finding out earlier in the morning I would not have to receive IV chemo today was relieving. But the thought of it would not leave my mind. Just two days before, I remembered the grand ole confrontation between the chemotherapy and me. It was getting old real fast, but I still had all but one week of the remaining 2.5 years. Looking forward to those days never happened; I looked forward to afterwards like a child looks forward to seeing his father come home from work. In an instant, everything would be right. Every pain would be nullified and life would be blissful. I remembered that life before wasn't as rosy as I was envisioning, but it would be on the other side of chemo for I knew that my perspective had blossomed into a richer understanding of healthy life, living it, and cherishing it.

I drifted off into sleep while waiting for the shuttle to return to the Ronald McDonald House. In my dream I greeted the nurse for the day and went through the rituals of prepping for infusion: pushing saline and heparin into the IV to ensure that it was not occluded. The heparin smelled sort of weird, but it was over shortly so it did not bother me considerably. I knew there were larger issues to worry about like the upcoming Vincristine and Daunomycine. She started a bag of fluids, as she departed to ensure the chemotherapy was acquired from the pharmacy. While I was being hydrated, mom and I chatted about my girlfriend, Jenny. Mom asked what I thought about her coming up that weekend to see me. I was pleased about the idea, but it still bothered me the conversation Jenny and I had the previous week. She had shared her opinion and confused state of mind in dating someone who had cancer and did not know if she could do it. Even though I said that I understood her position, I sure as hell did not. Nevertheless, I wanted to see her because teenage love is a silly thing and it was how I felt at the time.

The time was nearing again, as I saw the nurse return to the medicine room that she left minutes ago to retrieve my chemotherapy. She brought in numerous bags, and I knew that some were intended to be administered to me. It was no prize to receive these bags though, so it was disappointing. I took a deep breath, then another. I began talking to God in my mind, "Why? Please help me get through this round. Make it not as bad as Monday. I really don't want to feel bad, God. Is there any way you can help me out on this one? I promise I won't bother you again . . . until Friday." I smiled knowing that the prayer was ridiculous and that there was little stopping the upcoming treatment from nearly destroying my body and spirit.

Like Monday, the same drugs were given in combination. They were feared from the nausea that I was just beginning to get over from Monday's treatment, so these would likely just compile my level of nausea to new heights. I quickly learned that there is no maximum level of nausea; it can continue to increase forever. I watched the nurse connecting the bags, as I exhaled violently. The frustration was starting to take a toll on me; it was day three. I tried watching television and turning on my side to sleep, but it did not really matter what method I used—the results were always the same. I began to be overcome with nausea, seconds and minutes went by as I hoped the initial purging sensations would pass, but they never did.

I pointed to mom, which was code for "Give me the throw up bucket now." The reason I pointed was not indication of ugly intentions but instead it saved me from exerting effort from speaking. Talking to others while being nauseated was one of the things I grew to dislike. Two failed attempts at puking and then with the force of a Mack truck, I released the contents of my lunch and anything else that remained undigested from breakfast in one to two heaves. My body shook and jumped forward as the material exited my mouth and nose. The acidic substances burned my nasal cavities but there was nothing I could do to prevent it. My body wanted the substances out and it was clear that I had little control over what it felt was appropriate. Still, the nausea did not cease because I still had hours more of the chemotherapy drips. It was temporarily lessened but it was not 30 minutes later when the urge to vomit returned. This steady diet of purging and dry heaving continued not only during my visit in the medicine room but throughout the latter days following the chemo regiment. Chemotherapy effects are long-lasting; they affect cancer patients for durations of time just as medications for anxiety and depression but don't require the re-administrating of the medicine each day. In other words, even though the half-life of the medicine has passed, the effects are still felt on the body as they were in my case in particular. Learning this that week was mind-bendingly difficult. After this induction phase, I would be receiving chemotherapy once a week. Apparently, that meant that I would feel ill much more than just one day a week. More glorious news, so much I could barely wrap my mind around the notion of being sick for that long. Was it worth the battle that ensued for the chance of reaching wellness in the distant future?

My body was still nauseous, had nothing left in my stomach, and had barely enough energy to keep my eyes open for any amount of time. If one could imagine not eating for days, being deprived of liquids except the toxins fed into one's veins, and staring at the sun for hours while competing in a heavy-weight fight with chemotherapy, one could feel it firsthand. There was no chance of coming out on the other side of the treatment unscathed. I was just glad when I could be wheeled out of the medicine room to go back to the Ronald McDonald House. And then I awoke, as my mother tapped my shoulder saying, "The van is here." Wait a second; I was still in a daze. Had all that just happened? Apparently, it didn't. So even on a day in which I never received chemotherapy via IV injection, I had nightmares about it.

The waiting and sleeping throughout the day was wearing on my mind. It was not that I hated the hospital but after sitting there, lying there, and living there most of the day, it was time to go. Just seeing a wheelchair could draw up demons from my bellows, causing me to puke again and again, before becoming stable enough to depart the facility. I hadn't even received chemo that day, but I was still nauseous from Monday's long day. This tendency repeated itself two more times that night before finally I fell into slumber and out of consciousness.

Thursday

Mom was always my alarm clock, because I rarely heard the actual one go off. Whenever I did, I would not budge. Today, we had to hurry because it was later than we had normally woken up. Apparently, we were both fatigued from yesterday. We headed over to the hospital in order to eat something swiftly in the cafeteria to begin the day off on the right foot. Pancakes, hash browns, bacon, juice, and milk for me; Mom had her Diet Coke. Then, we headed over to assessment and triage for 9:00AM. By the time we arrived, there were many other patients already there. It was over 30 minutes before even completing the assessment and triage aspect of the day. Although waiting was not painful or nauseating, it was still inside the confines of the hospital. Being in hospitals for days on end will wear on anyone, especially the patient.

Following the A&T Clinic visit, mom and I walked back to the waiting area for my appointment in A Clinic, where I would be seen by Dr. Sandlund before getting my Asparaginase shot. Today, I lucked out in that I was called back only 10 minutes after waiting in that portion of the hospital. As a trade off, I did not see Dr. Sandlund. Instead, a nurse practitioner named Sandra introduced herself, telling me that she worked closely with Dr. Sandlund and would be conducting the examination this morning. She sensed I was disappointed and voiced her understanding since she agreed that Dr. Sandlund was the most impressive doctor with whom she has ever worked. After several minutes and the usual checks, she said that I looked to be doing well and handed me the daily numbers from my blood analysis, while asking what I had for breakfast. I informed her about the feast I had, which accounted for shifting my numbers to be high for certain markers. "No worries," she said. I was dismissed and sent to wait once more for the medicine room to call my name for my daily chemotherapy.

This was my second time that I would be receiving the Asparaginase shot, and upon entering the medicine room, I was more comfortable with the idea. It hurt badly on Tuesday, but it was nothing compared to the nausea with other chemo treatments. I became more observant of what was going on around me this time, since my nerves were calmed. As the nurse checked my bracelet identification tag to ensure that I was indeed Evan Ortlieb, I noticed the needle he was carrying. It was long and awfully large in gauge. The male nurse said that I needed to pull my pajama pants down. The nurse sprayed with analgesic spray on my leg, but I did not understand how that would be helpful when the spray was on the surface and the needle would be intramuscular. He held the shot in a fist like he was going to stab me with the needle like the guy in Alfred Hitchcock's *Psycho* (1960). No slow or gradual process here. It was a direct plunge into the quadriceps muscle. After being poked with the shot, I was required to check it twice before leaving the hospital. The first check was in 30 minutes, so I had to hang around in the medicine room. The nurse drew a circle on the muscle to mark where the shot had been given. Once he checked for a reaction and it looked fine, I was released to lunch but had to be back for the second check one hour later. He handed me a printout of my schedule for Saturday, the next time I would need to return to the hospital. This puzzled me. I thought that chemo would be administered during the work week; apparently, the regimens sometimes called for Saturday treatments. Learning about this upcoming Saturday prompted me to review the induction therapy schedule upon returning to my room later in the afternoon (see Figure 3). Meeting the needs of the patients was the number one priority, even before contemplating the strain and stresses it put on scheduling nurses and doctors at the hospital.

At lunch, mom had a turkey and Swiss cheese sandwich, and another Diet Coke. I ordered lasagna and broccoli—something slightly more substantial. Also, we were sure to grab some granola bars for in between meals later in the afternoon and evening. I had to get my money's worth of the free items. We went back to medicine room, and surprise, surprise, my leg checked out again fine. That's when mom coined the phrase, "Nappy time." "OK," I retorted. It sounded like she was talking to a two-year-old child. I was in fact her son so it did not bother me in the least. I just thought it was awkward sounding. Upon our return, the room was still cold and no light allowed inside, just the way I wanted it. I thought it was the perfect environment in which to attempt a nap. Even the smallest glimmers of life were shielded with taped curtains. We had the air conditioning on full force and the fans on high as well to drown out any noise that could emanate from the hallway, where children were playing. Any noise heard could awaken me because I

NHL 13
~~TOTAL XIIIB~~ - INDUCTION / CONSOLIDATION

Induction Therapy for 16085   EVAN ORTLIEB

Wk	Day 1	Day 2	Day 3	Day 4	Day 5	Day 6	Day 7
1	28Jun99 PRED VCR/DAUNO1 ITMHA 1#	29Jun99 PRED L-ASP 1	30Jun99 PRED	01Jul99 PRED L-ASP2	02Jul99 PRED	03Jul99 PRED L-ASP3	04Jul99 PRED

Wk	Day 8	Day 9	Day 10	Day 11	Day 12	Day 13	Day 14
2	05Jul99 PRED VCR/DAUNO2 L-ASP 4	06Jul99 PRED	07Jul99 PRED L-ASP 5	08Jul99 PRED	09Jul99 PRED L-ASP 6	10Jul99 PRED	11Jul99 PRED

Wk	Day 15	Day 16	Day 17	Day 18	Day 19	Day 20	Day 21
3	12Jul99 PRED VCR 3 TMP/SMZ ~~BMA*~~	13Jul99 PRED TMP/SMZ	14Jul99 PRED TMP/SMZ	15Jul99 PRED TMP/SMZ	16Jul99 PRED TMP/SMZ	17Jul99 PRED TMP/SMZ	18Jul99 PRED TMP/SMZ

Wk	Day 22	Day 23	Day 24	Day 25	Day 26	Day 27	Day 28
4	19Jul99 PRED VCR 4 VP/ARAC 1 ITMHA 2# TMP/SMZ +-BMA**-	20Jul99 PRED TMP/SMZ	21Jul99 PRED TMP/SMZ	22Jul99 PRED VP/ARAC 2 TMP/SMZ	23Jul99 PRED TMP/SMZ	24Jul99 PRED TMP/SMZ	25Jul99 PRED TMP/SMZ

Wk	Day 29	Day 30	Day 31	Day 32	Day 33	Day 34	Day 35
5	26Jul99 STOP PRED VP/ARAC 3 TMP/SMZ	27Jul99 TMP/SMZ	28Jul99 TMP/SMZ	29Jul99 TMP/SMZ	30Jul99 TMP/SMZ	31Jul99 TMP/SMZ	01Aug99 TMP/SMZ

Wk	Day 36	Day 37	Day 38	Day 39	Day 40	Day 41	Day 42
6	02Aug99 TMP/SMZ	03Aug99 TMP/SMZ	04Aug99 TMP/SMZ	05Aug99 TMP/SMZ	06Aug99 TMP/SMZ	07Aug99 TMP/SMZ	08Aug99 TMP/SMZ

Wk	Day 43	Day 44	Day 45	Day 46	Day 47	Day 48	Day 49
7	09Aug99 ITMHA 3# BMA	10Aug99 HDMTX#1 6MP	11Aug99 6MP	12Aug99 6MP	13Aug99 6MP	14Aug99 6MP	15Aug99 6MP

Wk	Day 50	Day 51	Day 52	Day 53	Day 54	Day 55	Day 56
8	16Aug99 6MP	17Aug99 HDMTX#2 6MP ITMHA 4	18Aug99 6MP	19Aug99 6MP	20Aug99 6MP	21Aug99 6MP	22Aug99 6MP

Wk	Day 57						
9	23Aug99 6MP						

1st day of remission

Post consol

1st day of remission

post remission

* BMA on day 15, if pt has >= 5% blasts, pts on low risk
protocol will be moved to high risk.
** BMA is performed on day 29 only if ANC < 300.
Note: Patients with CNS leukemia at DX or blasts in the CSF
should receive two additional ITMHA on days 8 and 15.
2ml CSF to PK for asparagine

Figure 3. Non-Hodgkin's Lymphoma Protocol 13.

153

was a soft-sleeper so these preventive measures were fully logical. The room resembled a cave, dark and closed off, to escape from everything else. The nap lasted from 2:30-5:00 or so.

I woke up, noticing that mom was only half-way asleep. She was even a lighter sleeper than me. It had more to do with being at my beck and call, and willing to do whatever it took to bring me any kind of comfort during this trying time. I asked mom if she could make me some eggs and biscuits downstairs. It took her 45 seconds before she headed out the door, downstairs, and ready to cook. Her efforts were surely taken for granted, but her assistance was not only necessary but unmatched by anyone else during the treatment period of my life.

As it turned out, a church group was cooking dinner but I didn't feel well enough to go to the sociable occasion. The group prepared salad, rolls, and chicken casserole with tetrazzini. Mom ate a bit downstairs before she came back upstairs with the food. The volunteers sent up their thoughts and prayers with mom since I was feeling ill, and they hoped the food would provide some nourishment. When Mom came back to the room, I didn't feel like eating right away. Thirty minutes later, I started eating some and finished about half of it. One would think that would be the end of the day, but being a teenage boy, I became hungry again later that night. It was not practical to request some food from Mom, so I asked if I could go downstairs to find something to snack on. She said that she would join me, so she got dressed. In contrast, I did not care what I looked like and was perfectly content wearing my pajamas that I had on. Throughout the Ronald McDonald House, to the hospital, or even around town, I wore my pajamas. We went downstairs and raided the shared pantry, finding some cereal and candy, preparing it before bringing it up to the room, which of course was against the rules. I took a shower shortly later, which made me feel fresher than expected. And soon I dove into bed for the night at 9:30PM.

Friday

Loafing around is the perfect descriptor of what my goals were for Friday. Waking up around 10:30AM and lying in bed for awhile longer was just what the doctor ordered. I went to urinate twice and crashed back in bed before eventually getting up for the day at 11:15AM. Mom was just as content as I was with doing nothing. Busy weeks of sitting in the hospital at various waiting areas took any desire to be active completely away and this was just day five. Even though we could do anything we so desired, we desired to do absolutely nothing. The day was free for us.

It was clear that I needed to eat something soon, because I was supposed to take medication with each meal. With it being 11:15AM already, lunch would be pushed back a few hours but nothing with which to be overly concerned. I allowed Mom to take her shower first, because she was a woman who took several minutes to get prepped, dressed, and ready for the day. Her attire and dress were always superior to any of the others, and I would not have it any other way. It set my mother apart—her gentle presence and selflessness made her quintessentially unique in my eyes.

Pancakes! How could I have forgotten one of my favorite breakfast dishes that mom cooked? Those little pancakes with the ridge of crispiness, ahh, were just what I sought. I could taste them before the batter was even prepared. "What do you think, Mom? I am kind of feeling some pancakes today." "Whatever you want Ev," she responded. Those words held true for she would and did do everything in her power to appease me and reduce the stress on my body. I just struggled relaying my wishes and thoughts to her while I was in constant nausea. This state of paralysis, being under constant duress from chemotherapy, caused both my body and mind to be less sharp. Still, the pancakes would provide me with some level of temporary happiness and the sooner they came out, the better. There they came with syrup and butter lying atop the three pancakes on the large white plate, never stacked, but instead spread out.

Without waiting another second, I dug the fork that I had been holding for at least five minutes into one of them. I ate two of the pancakes and in doing so, realized that they tasted different. I was puzzled because mom's pancakes always tasted the same— moist and lightly cooked. These were bland and without any flavor. I jumped up to speak with mom, who was just on the other side of the kitchen entrance. Leaving the dining area for a moment, I found Mom and inquired about the pancakes. She was surprised to hear my critique, but took the blame for inadequately preparing them to my liking. Still, the mystery persisted. What was the deal with the pancakes? Mom came out to where I was sitting and tried a bite of the remaining pancake. She chewed while reflecting on its taste. Her conclusion was that it tasted the same as always. "No way!," I said. Was she right? She could not possibly know what she was talking about because who would know my taste buds better than me? I grabbed my prednisone pill and a glass of milk next to my plate and finished them off right away. I was disappointed in not only how breakfast tasted but of how my body was changing to my disliking.

After telling Mom I was going to the teen room to play pool, I briskly walked towards the elevator like never before since arriving in Memphis. I was not calm. How on earth could food taste differently now? Did chemotherapy really affect every aspect of my life? Entering the teen room it became clearer that the answer was yes. No one was around. Many of the patients received treatments on Fridays, but this week I was not scheduled for any. Standing in the room, hitting the balls with more voracity than normal, I stood looking around, walking in circles, pacing, and thinking—I am all alone. I have no friends here. My mother is looking out for me and doing whatever she can, but I have no one else with whom to speak, converse, and engage in causal friendship. There were people who came and went, but no true friends. It was the lack of connections made that began to tatter my mental framework. I did not feel close to the others there nor my friends and family back in Baton Rouge. There was a unique place where I was and no one else was there with me. Loneliness began to settle in and it was a very new feeling for me, having grown up in a modest house with siblings who were a part of everything I did. This journey was to be different and I did not like how it was developing. I left the teen room just as fast as I came in and with the same negative demeanor.

Walking back to my room, using the keycard to gain access to the room, and sitting on the bed followed. Mom was certainly curious asking me, "What is the matter?" The ever-common "nothing" was my response. I did not want to discuss my feelings. It was not becoming of a male adolescent or at least not to me, so I buried my thoughts in my sheets once again. I told mom I was tired, but it was not why I was going back to bed. She knew better too. One thing was stated on the surface but the underlying reasoning was very clear to my mom—the only other person who could at least in some way understand my feelings.

By 2:00pm, I was becoming incredibly hungry, which had grown by the minute since my unsatisfactory breakfast. Several other families were around the shared kitchen area of the Ronald McDonald House when we went downstairs to find something to eat for lunch. Meeting others while eating was a regular event, since it was still the first week of my elongated stay in Memphis. As we began looking around the pantry to gather ideas for a meal, my mother met another mother and son. Introducing me to the woman, my mother spoke with his mother who pointed to a 17-year-old male named Darren. When I looked at him, all I saw was his big face. I prayed that it would never happen to me . . . thank God because he looked terrible. He looked like someone who ate 24 hours a day nonstop. His cheeks were bloated, had a big belly, and had substantial arms and legs. I thought that his reactions to the drugs were abnormal until I saw two others the same day with a similar appearance. They said it had to do with the Dexamethasone he was taking. Interestingly enough, I was on the same medication but showed no symptoms like he did. Speaking with his mother, she said that Darren had not suffered any changes too until he had been taking them for two weeks. He was finishing his third week at the time.

As I sat at the table eating, I looked at my schedule of medications, noticing that I was supposed to take one with my lunch that day. I found it in my mom's purse, checked the label, and noticed that it was the same medicine that was making Darren so hungry and heavy—Dexamethasone. OK, I thought. Cheers to getting fat. I sarcastically joked with myself and popped the pill with my meal. Dear God, don't let me get fat. Growing up I had always been as skinny as a twig and could never envision myself differently. I was already looking differently in terms of tiredness and color of my skin, but I still felt that Dexamethasone could not possibly have the same effects on me as it did the other cancer patients.

Eating with some others was more enjoyable than eating alone. I did not feel nauseous any more, which played a significant role in level of sociability and my enjoyment of the food before me. Talking to Darren was fascinating because he was the first cancer patient with whom I had a thorough conversation. He spoke about his tough experiences, but held a positive twist on them by thanking the Lord for still being here on earth. Seeing his refusal to let his cancer and the chemotherapy get to him was refreshing. What was difficult for him was living in Memphis. He came from Nebraska, where his family was primarily self-sufficient from what they raised on their farm. It did not take me long to have the pleasure of tasting his mother's seven course meals that she continued to prepare for

Darren at the Ronald McDonald House. His mother was a blessing to him, just as mine was for me.

Once my late lunch was finished, I walked to the lounging room adjacent to the dining room to watch some television. Of course nothing was on during the daytime that was worth viewing in my opinion, so I departed to my room. Besides, I was sick of watching television in general. It was just that think-free activities were easier to experience than those that required mental function.

Mom and I talked for awhile about Darren's family. Their strength gave us promise for how we would deal with the coming weeks of chemotherapy during my induction phase of my treatment at St. Jude. Referring to her cooking and positive temperament, "How does she do it?," mom asked. "I don't know . . . but she is one of the kindest women I have ever met," I said. Darren's mother had no worries, placing her total trust in the Lord to bring her son healing. That seemed so hard for us to envision, since I was hurting so badly most days and it was just days ago that I learned of my life-changing diagnosis. I could not envision having such a positive mindset, especially when her son looked so different from his customary appearance. In a swollen figure, Darren suffered just as I did, but maintained an exemplary attitude towards doing what was necessary to get his life back in order. Having realized that Darren and I were clearly on different levels, had different types of cancer, and different chemotherapy regiments, I did the only natural thing— felt selfish momentarily and drowned my sorrows in the bed once again.

That Friday night, I did not leave the room even though my body was not nauseated. I was in a state of confusion. I felt lows like never before in my life, and the highs were not occurring anymore. Meeting new people, playing pool, sleeping in sometimes, and not having to complete school work may sound like every teenager's dream, but for me, they were just aspects of my living with cancer in Memphis. I began to hate it. My attitude was shifting more negatively because of my isolation from my known world in Baton Rouge, LA. I did not want to eat dinner or socialize with the other families. My mother recommended that I call some family members in Baton Rouge to tell them how things are going. I declined for the night, saying that I would do that tomorrow. The end of the day could not come soon enough, so I crashed in bed at 8:00PM for the night.

Saturday

My first thoughts upon waking up were related to chemo. It was Saturday for crying out loud, but the schedule once again called for an Asparaginase shot and prednisone to be taken by mouth. Even though it was frustrating, I did not fear them because neither medication made me nauseated so it was more bothersome that anything. It was great that this would be a nausea-free treatment because I was just starting to feel free from the effects of my Monday long day of chemo. Two days of no nausea this week came none too soon. I had high hopes for this weekend. Too bad it had to start off with a trip to the hospital.

Breakfast was also much more enjoyable without fearing that it would be viewed again in an hour exiting my orifices. Mom suggested that I try some eggs and biscuits with jelly. Oooh, it sounded tasty, just like she used to make for me during my childhood when she was still living with me at home. I sunk my teeth into the biscuit after spooning some jelly between the layers. I steadily ate four of the six biscuits and three scrambled eggs without hesitation. Mom said she was not hungry, so I did not bother saving her any eggs at all—yet another example of putting my wants and

164

needs first. My mother prepared this breakfast and then hurried afterwards to get ready for the shuttle ride to the hospital. I took my time eating, knowing that I would be going dressed as is, without concern for my appearance. They were going to see me look worse off when I was nauseated and my appearance was not anything to be proud of anyway. Off we went to the hospital for my third intramuscular Asparaginase shot.

Being the only ones on the shuttle felt awkward. Of course no other children had chemotherapy on Saturday. Perhaps they had in the past, but I was trying to find something with which to pout. Being miserable for long durations makes one feel sorry for himself. After entering the hospital, I checked in and was actually able to socialize with the staff inside. Most other days my nausea caused me to keep speaking to a minimum. Maybe that is partially why I talk all day long as an educator today.

With my mood improved from conversing with others, I completed my blood work, as the nurse commented on my upbeat demeanor. I told her that I was not nauseated and it was reason enough to have a smile on my face. Proceeding quickly to the waiting area, I asked mom if she had the book I had begun a week ago. Luckily she had it in her enormous purse, one of those ones that are all decked out. The book, *Tiger Woods: The Makings of a Champion* (1997), was given to me by some of my father's co-workers. They knew I was an avid golfer and thought that I would enjoy reading it in my lengthy periods of waiting at the hospital. Thank God for it; it let me dream. Reading about Tiger Woods' flight to success reassured me that anything was possible—from golfing accomplishments to defeating diseases.

Within minutes my name was called to go inside the medicine room. This was the shortest waiting time yet; perhaps, it had something to do with the fact that no one else was scheduled to receive chemo that day. I digress. To my surprise I saw most of the same nurses who were there the weekend I arrived in Memphis. This was the weekend crew, I found out later. They worked Friday, Saturday, and Sunday 12 hours a day. Not too bad for a work week in my opinion. They were also more relaxed than the other crews, which fit my personality better. Having no worries was what I was shooting for when in the medicine room and they aimed to please. Ron was my nurse for this injection. Instead of giving me some lines about how much it was going to hurt and so on, he said, "You're a grown man. You can handle this little shot. No big deal." His statements were spot on. There was nothing to fear regarding these Asparaginase shots, at least not from my previous two experiences. I think my personality today reflects that which Ron displayed that summer of 1999. I find myself telling students and others alike that some things just have to be done. We will knock it out and move on, so there is no need to worry because worrying has never done anything to help the situation. Matter of fact, this is yet another example of something my father taught me throughout childhood and reaffirms even today.

The shot was prepared and readied to be given. Like in a nightmarish fashion, Ron stood tall in front of me. The overhead light shined over his shoulder and into my strained eyes. He raised the needle, squirting the liquid out of the needle so as to release any air bubbles that might be present. Then, Ron sat on his swivel stool and said, "On three. One, two, (stick). Just as the previous times, the insertion of the liquid into my muscle burned as if my body was rejecting the foreign substance. It felt awful, but at the same time, it was over. The pain was there, yes, but I was still nausea free. That feeling cannot be topped for a cancer patient undergoing chemotherapy. I sat in the reclined chair for 30 minutes before getting up and walking around a bit. Mom asked if I wanted to go to lunch. This time, though, I just wanted to get back to reading the book about Tiger Woods. He was an icon with which I held in high regard and keeping him on my mind served to motivate and simultaneously distract me from worrying about pain, loneliness, and other burdens I was holding. The only issue that arose was about 40 minutes into the one hour of time I was trying to fill, my eyes began to tire. I handed mother the text, telling her about my eyes. I just relaxed, set my head back, and waited another 20 minutes or so until Ron came back to check on me. He looked at the leg, as it appeared to be normal and free of any adverse reactions. Telling him about my eyes tiring, he did not sound surprised. Ron spoke about how it was a very regular occurrence, and that most children recognized it upon playing video games. I suppose that it was not a big deal, relatively speaking, but just something else to add to the plight of my once in shape and healthy body.

After waiting over an hour in the medicine room once the shot was given, mom and I decided to check out the city. Everyone spoke about how great Beale Street was, likening it to Bourbon

Street in New Orleans. Well, if it was anything like Bourbon Street, I was not interested in seeing it. Drunks galore . . . count me out. I did not want to spend my few moments of nausea-free living amongst crowds of people. Instead we drove down the two streets we heard about where there were attractions, places to dine, and so on. Poplar Avenue and Union Avenue were our destinations. All we had to do now was find them.

We drove out of the hospital parking lot and turned left twice, like the gate attendant suggested we do. That road led directly to Poplar, so we drove down and stayed on Poplar until we found something that drew our interest. All we saw at first were pawn shops, gas stations, and bail bondsmen locations. It said a lot about the location to have those as the most popular businesses in the area. Heading towards midtown we passed several neighborhoods, a golf course, which interested me, and a small college. Then, we saw three attractions near one another: a bookstore, Piccadilly—the restaurant, and a movie theatre. Since we were not yet hungry, we chose to visit the bookstore, particularly because my mom was a fervent reader and I was finishing the one book I had in my possession in Memphis.

From the outside of the building, the bookstore looked rather small by my standards. However upon our entrance, I realized that it was larger than I had assumed. The organization style of this and every bookstore for that matter always amused me, as it was impossible to find the area you are looking for without asking a sales clerk, like looking in the dictionary for the spelling of a word with which you do not know how to spell. Nevertheless, I walked in between all the aisles noticing the genres of texts, finding the magazines in the rear. These interested me more than most books for a variety of reasons, like my short attention span and difficulties focusing while waiting in loud lobbies and noisy medicine rooms. Meanwhile, mom said she would be looking for some crossword and cryptogram paperbacks. I did not think anything about her statement at first, but shortly later, I considered as to why she was looking for something other than the fiction novels with which she loved. The primary motive was that just like me, she found it difficult to concentrate for durations in the environments in which we lived at the hospital and at the Ronald McDonald House. I did not assist in her pursuit of her reading interests by mandating that there be little to no light in our room. Sleep, nappy times, and overly chilled temperatures created the worst possible reading space. It never entered my mind though.

Walking from right to left in front of the magazines, I realized that there were hundreds of magazines that the bookstore carried. From provocative to children-oriented, I kept looking for the sports magazines, even though the woman on one of them caught my eye. I wondered why they put her on the cover. Then I came across sporting magazines that were generic, and then others that were specific sports-related like GOLF Magazine. I thumbed through a couple of them before grabbing ESPN-The Magazine. I sat on one of the benches next to someone else reading a magazine. I did not know what I was looking for specifically, but just curious as to what was happening in the sports world. In my childhood, I watched SportsCenter in the mornings before school so as to stay abreast of the sporting world each day. Nerdy as it may be, it interested me because I had an array of sports pursuits. About 15 minutes after sitting down, my mom came by to check on me. I do not blame her. We were in a city with which neither of us knew much about and we had never been in the bookstore before either. I said I was doing fine, but was growing somewhat hungry. "Five more minutes," I

171

said. She agreed and went to return the books to the shelf. I finished reading an article that reflected on Mark McGwire's home run record setting year in 1998. I found mom back near the center of the store and inquired why she was not going to purchase the word search book. She said that she just did not want to for whatever reason. "OK, let's roll out of here," I said. Knowing that Piccadilly, which was a favorite restaurant of mine for its home-style cooking, was across the street, we proceeded to eat dinner there.

Finding fried catfish, rice and gravy, fried okra, and a sweet roll, I was looking forward to sitting down and feasting on the first meal in a legitimate restaurant this week. I tasted the fish and then my fried okra. The verdict did not take long to issue—it was not like southern Louisiana cooking. "Where is the taste?," I asked sarcastically. Mom said that she figured we were not that much north of Louisiana, but apparently it made a difference. The food was good, do not get me wrong, it just lacked the seasoning and rich flavors that had accompanied me throughout my 16 years of residence in Louisiana. That is when mom stated, "Maybe it has something to do with your treatments? Here, let me taste it." Was it again a result of my receiving chemotherapy and it affecting my taste buds like before? In part it probably was, however, the food in front of me did not have much seasoning, as mom quickly assured me after tasting it for herself. The taste though did not stop me from devouring my choices of food. My appetite was high because I remained nausea free. Therefore, I was going to get my nourishment while I could because Monday would be here before I knew it. As I was finishing the meal, the manager came by and introduced himself, ensuring that we had a great experience at his location. My mother explained that we were new to the area because of my recent diagnosis. Piccadilly was already on the list of restaurants that accepted St. Jude vouchers so most of our meal would be paid for by the hospital. The manager asked what kind of dessert I wanted. I declined at first, but after prying a bit further, I decided on an all-time favorite—lemon ice box pie. The pecan pie came to mind, but again, I did not want to risk something that is a southern tradition. Returning to the table, he brought out my piece of pie and assured that it was on the house. He also gave my mother a to-go cup of sweetened tea. He was very kind, making up for the food not meeting my expectations.

We left the restaurant and drove to the other side of the parking lot to see what movies were playing at the theatre. There were none that jumped off the billboard and caught our eye, so we drove off, figuring that we could decide tomorrow if seeing a movie was of any interest. After all, things change daily around here and who knows how I would be feeling then? Mom and I arrived back at the Ronald McDonald House, entering the building and walking into our room. There was no better way to finish off our day than to quickly ready for bed. And so, we did just that. I jumped into bed and it felt great. Off to sleep I went, quickly this time, thanks again to being nausea free for an entire day.

Sunday

Sunday morning came and as I woke up, an eerie feeling came over me. I wiped my eyes, trying to open them. Then as I somehow made it to the bathroom without the assistance of sight, I realized that I was still free from feelings of nausea. I did not know whether to be elated or scared. Sure, tomorrow would soon be here, but I had a whole day with which to feel good once again. It was the first time that I could plan an entire day. Just as those thoughts entered my mind, I saw that the clock said it was 8:47AM. This

174

prompted me to make the executive decision of immediately getting back into the bed and sleeping.

Waking from my slumber some two hours later, I figured I should get out of bed and find something to eat. Mom was still lying in bed because she did not want to leave me alone in case I needed her for something. Sleeping for the amount of time I did would easily cause a healthy person to become depressed. What was there to live for? More sleep. It did not seem like an inviting offer to spend time with me there, but I was surely grateful for the assistance she supplied me. "Mom, you don't have to cook for me this morning. Besides, it is almost lunch already." She said that would be fine. Neither of us especially wanted to get dressed up just to walk to the kitchen so we did not. Hunting through one of the pantries, we found some pop tarts and individually packed cereal containers. I grabbed two cereal boxes and a package of Pop Tarts. She grabbed one cereal box and some milk from the refrigerator. That morning was our first breakfast together. Other families were around, but I was more focused on having a conversation with my mother about everything that was going on, including my girlfriend saying that she would try to drive to Memphis the following weekend, my father and brother trying to stay updated on my ongoings, and my younger sister who still did not fully understand the level of severity of my cancer diagnosis. Handling these family issues was a hardship that came with the territory. Luckily, whichever parent of mine was not with me at the time, was handling those other matters to minimize the stress on each other. Their teamwork, even though they were divorced, proved an ever-important aspect of the complexity of undergoing chemotherapy.

As we finished our lunchtime meal, mom and I debated about what we should do throughout the afternoon and evening. I was not sure yet, so I decided to think it over while playing some pool in the teen room. Mom was not a pool shark, so she opted out. This was perfectly acceptable because we both needed some personal space, since we were with one another virtually 24 hours a day for over a week. I went into the teen room and to my dismay, there were eight and nine year olds playing with the pool cues. Slapping the balls around like they were playing with marbles, it wore on my patience. I was not the type of fellow who would barge in, take the cues, and tell them to get lost, although I did consider it. I waited impatiently until I asked if I could have a try and they agreed. Apparently, I had not made myself perfectly clear though. The children thought I was saying I wanted to play against them, without rules, slapping the balls into the holes by dragging them against the cue until they went into the pockets. Within five minutes of its commencement, I handed the cue back to one of them, as I had my fill of playing with ignorant children for the day. There I was on my one free day and I could not enjoy myself in the teen room for God's sake. It was back to my room.

The children in the teen room had gotten me so sidetracked that I forgot to consider what I wanted to do for the rest of the day, besides remain free of overenthusiastic and energetic children. My mother understood my frustrations because children wore on her patience levels too. I had already forgotten that I was free of nausea. There I was complaining about not being able to play pool when in hindsight, it was the best day of the week as far as how I felt physically. Talking some more with Mom, we soon realized that we did not know of much to do in Memphis. We heard about people going to Graceland, riding on the paddleboats on the Mississippi River, putt putt golf across the river in Arkansas, and going to the mall in Germantown. Yet none of those were interesting to me that day. I had already become accustomed to just hanging out and staying low key. It is the constant feelings of nausea that solidify these feelings within cancer patients. Still I held other feelings like "I have to get out of here!" So eventually, we chose to get directions and head towards the mall in Germantown, Tennessee, not because we wanted to buy something in particular but because we wanted to get out of the Ronald McDonald House. We felt cooped up all week long.

Navigating the interstates proved to be somewhat more daunting than expected. Even though there were two interstate roads that met in our hometown of Baton Rouge, there were several in Memphis like I-55 and 240 that included a loop around the city with which we were unfamiliar. After making one minor error, we were headed in the proper direction. About 20 minutes later, we exited the interstate system in Germantown, noticing that things were very different from downtown Memphis. Apparently, Memphis was a sprawling city and this was one of the suburbs, because it had numerous high-end restaurants and a relatively new looking mall. While we were parking, we saw a sign depicting that there was a movie theatre inside. We thought that this too would be nicer than the one we saw the day before in midtown. We entered the building in the food court and continued for awhile. I went into one of the gaming stores while mom headed into Banana Republic. Browsing around, I had nothing in mind that I was looking for, not to mention I was not interested in buying anything. Our trip's purpose was just to leave the Ronald McDonald House for some time and enjoy my full day of being nausea free.

 I walked back towards where my mother was perusing. She too was not really looking to buy anything, so we agree to grab a bite to eat in the food court. The choice was easy—Chinese all the way. We ordered some mixed plates of sesame chicken, sweet and sour chicken, fried rice, and vegetables. I filled my belly to the limit because I did not know when the next time I would have the opportunity. While walking to the opposite side of the mall, I concluded that it was no different from any other mall I had seen, except for the inside-the-mall movie theatre. Still, it did not have any movies playing that appealed to me so we headed back to downtown Memphis an hour later. On the ride back, my stomach sent signals to my brain indicating, "Perhaps, you ate too much Chinese food." Nevertheless, I was able to hold out until getting back to our room, where my food selection and quantity ran its course through my body.

The rest of the day consisted of eating a light meal for dinner and a snack before bed, because I knew that I would have to fast the following day until after receiving blood work. Mom and I hung out mostly in the room, reading some and catching an occasional shut eye. While eating dinner, we watched television downstairs to stay current with the outside world. I spoke with my father on the telephone that night and I recognized how badly he felt that he could not be with me every second of the day in Memphis. He was working in Baton Rouge and had only so many weeks off each year. I told him how well I was currently feeling, and refrained from talking about my fears for the upcoming weeks ahead. Some things were better off left unsaid, until now.

Chapter 7:

Damn, These People are Crazy!

Life-challenging events like cancer diagnosis and treatment change lives. Perspectives are reshaped and structured accordingly. This is one of the reasons why I am grateful for having been diagnosed with cancer. My views and feelings on issues are unique, which is beneficial but also isolating. Sure, I maintain a refined focus on those things that actually matter in life without worrying about trivial details, but I am also separated from remembering and understanding common perceptions. Most people are not content each day with just being alive. Most people do not thank God for not being hurt daily. Most people do not treat their bodies with total attention and precaution. It is not that doing these acts is wrong, because it is not so. It is proper in every way, but it draws a dividing line between those who have had these experiences and those who had not.

Sometimes, people tell me that my sentiments and expressed feelings are judgmental. Although I take pride in being a Christian, it hurts me dearly to see others abuse each other or even themselves. Most times, there is nothing that I can do about it, so why worry? I do not have an answer for that dilemma but I can say that when it affects an innocent child, I have a big problem with it. One of my students recently quoted me as saying, "There is one thing in life that you don't screw up and that is a kid." My personal connection with pediatric cancer patients leads me to share the following stories with you about their mistreatment.

There are four events in which I will never forget and I hope that you do not either. In order to fully explain these issues, I must paint a picture for you to survey. The accounts are very real and graphic in content and in the language used to express my sentiments.

The dynamic duo

A teenage girl, appearing to be approximately 16 years old, and her mother exited the front doors of St. Jude Children's Research Hospital. It was obvious that the teenager was a patient; she had no hair on her head, an IV taped to her arm, and a blue identification bracelet that patients must wear at all times on the premises. She likely had some type of treatment to complete later in the day. The mother and daughter headed towards one of the benches outside to sit down and relax for awhile, much like I had already done. Watching with my knees spread out and slouched on the bench, I gazed towards them. The sun was shining so it was hard to keep my eyes completely open. They began chatting with one another, just like any other mother-daughter pair. It was pleasing to see that they were in good spirits on their break from the long day at the hospital.

Being bald, the same age of the girl, and a cancer patient, there was only one obvious difference between the two of us—the fortitude to which we displayed in our efforts to combat the cancer within our bodies. While I was trying to get a breath of fresh air, she and her mother were lighting up their cigarettes, polluting both the air inside and outside of what once was precious. I had to stop and think. Let me get this straight. There is a girl who is obviously undergoing chemotherapy treatments, and she is smoking! Not only that, but her mother is doing the same preposterous thing right beside her. I thought that the hospital was wasting its time fighting a disease that would most likely make itself known at a later date. What a waste of life, or two for that matter. Thanks for being a great role model, mom. You should be proud.

A world away

In the underground garage of the hospital, patients who were having procedures and trips to the medicine room were allowed to park for easy entrance into the hospital. After finding a parking spot in the rear of the lot, I walked back towards the entry doors. About half-way, I noticed a 10-year-old child sitting in a wheelchair. Due to avascular necrosis, many of St. Jude's cancer patients must rely on crutches and wheelchairs to navigate the grounds. This sick 10-year-old boy was slumped over from apparently feeling extremely nauseous. It was miserable just seeing the condition of the boy; I cannot even fathom what he felt like at the time. He kept making groaning noises, likely from the pain he was enduring. Was there something that I could do to help him?

As I approached the boy, I saw that he was not alone. Just a foot away but yet on a different planet, his mother sat in an indoor smoking facility. Inside, there were several people smoking; although it was ventilated, it appeared as if the smoke could be cut with a knife. With her back turned to the boy, she socialized with others inside the room laughing. All the while, her son sat on the other side of the Plexiglas desperately wanting his mother to take him home. "In a minute," she said, turning half-way around to project her voice towards her son.

Was this actually happening? Was this mother telling her chronically ill son that he needed to be patient for she had a social event that took priority with which she directed her attention? I stared at this pathetic excuse for a life and thought: your child is exhausted, longs to lie down, and nauseated beyond comprehension; meanwhile, you just intensify his agony. You do not deserve to be a mother. By not meeting the needs of your sick child, you clearly demonstrate just how despicable you are. One day will come when you will be judged on your actions and for your sake, I hope for pity. In actuality, you deserve nothing more or less than to be hooked up intravenously to receive high doses of chemotherapy while having doctors ignore your begging and pleading for assistance. Only then could you possibly have a clue as to what your son must deal with on a regular basis. Good riddance.

Death breath

In the third short story, and maybe the most graphic of the four, an elderly grandmother, probably in her late-sixties, cares for a young child approximately one year old. Because the mother was nowhere close-by, the grandmother watched over the child. She held the baby like any loving parent/grandparent would, cradling him in her arms. Socializing with other family members, it seemed like they were having a pleasant time in the accompaniment of one another.

The child was a cancer patient, as he had a mask with which he was supposed to wear to protect him from harmful airborne pathogens in the air from foreign particles like those emanating from the construction work that was going on. This neutropenic child had an immune system that could not easily fight off infections; thus, his caretakers were supposed to be extremely cautious. When children are in this condition, they cannot even eat cooked foods from restaurants or even leftovers because of the possibility of the food becoming tainted. Unfortunately, this child's mask was hanging from his neck. It was not on his face, which under certain circumstances could be understood. To top it off, this grandmother was smoking a cigarette (a.k.a. cancer stick) and blowing her exhaled toxins into her grandson's face, while saying, "he doesn't look too good today" to the others around. Hello! You are the dumbest person on earth if you think that he should feel fine when you are killing him with your callous behavior. Are you really that uneducated and ignorant? It does not take a genius to figure out what you are doing is not helping his health. Instead of approaching the woman and having a knockdown confrontation, I took an alternate method. I allowed her to continue to kill herself. I just hope the innocent child lived.

At all costs

The final scenario involves a mother and daughter with whom my family befriended. Katie and her mother, Karen, regularly associated with us at the hospital. However, they did not stay at the Ronald McDonald House because they were kicked out for breaking regulations- those that prohibited individuals from smoking while inside their personal room. Every hour or two, her mother made statements like: "Ahhh, I'm just so worried about her . . . I need a smoke break." Indeed, she did need a break . . . of something over her head. She could not look past her own selfish pursuits of getting a fix to realize that she was pawning off her very young daughter (around four years old or so) on someone to care for while she smoked outside. Her other option was to just smoke next to her, which she did in those instances when no one would help her. Awh, poor thing. Although her behavior was ludicrous, it did not come close to the audacity of what followed.

While Karen and Katie stayed at the Wyndham Hotel in downtown Memphis, paid for by St. Jude, at a rate around $100 per night, Karen broke the rules of the hotel too. St. Jude had an agreement with the hotel to reserve two floors, maintaining these as forever smoke-free zones so as to ensure healthy environments for patients when they stayed in Memphis. Karen called my mother one evening from the hotel while we were residing at the Ronald McDonald House. She asked if my mother could take her to the convenience store down the road to pick up some juice for Katie. Without question, my mother said, "Of course." Mom would never consider anything more important than caring for children. I agreed to watch Katie so they could go without disturbing the child. She was so cute and lovable. After meeting Karen at the entrance of the hotel, she and my mother departed heading towards the store. Karen went inside and exited the building a couple of minutes later with only one product- her pack of cigarettes.

"What about the juice?," inquired mom. My mother was disgusted. "That's what you needed?" Karen concurred, using the excuse, "Well, I knew if I told you it was for a pack of cigarettes, you would not have done it." You think? That is not the end of the story though. Returning to the hotel, Karen invited my mother upstairs to their room. Upon entering the room, my mother immediately noticed how the room wreaked of cigarette smoke, like a cloud of smoke hitting you in the face. Instead of denying it this time though, like she had done at the Ronald McDonald House, Karen explained that she kept the 'do not disturb' sign on the outside of the door for their entire stay and shoved towels underneath the door to block any remnants of smoke from seeping out of the room. She thought she was crafty for figuring out how to temporarily not get caught smoking in the room. Was this third grade? Was she really resorting to excuses for not getting caught with her hand in the cookie jar? Indeed, her practice was temporarily successful in doing what she wanted as well as keeping the smoke in her baby's lungs.

I saw Karen and Katie in the summer of 2008 at the Memphis Grizzly House, a short-term facility used by St. Jude patients, when I returned to St. Jude for an annual check-up. I recognized the mother right away; she had not changed much, while Katie was 12 years old and looked totally different. Within the first three minutes of our conversation, the mother became antsy and said, "You don't smoke, do you?" I had nothing to say and simply shook my head. "Well, I have to go smoke . . . we just got in from the plane ride," said Karen. Her daughter followed her outside as she did years before. "Oh," said Karen, "We are staying in room 2014 . . . you should come hang out." I think it is obvious that I did not go to their room. That was the last conversation we had; just as well, because I have nothing to say to her other than I cannot wait for your daughter to be out of your house and on her own for her future is bright despite years of abuse.

Chapter 8:

Missing It All

Moving away from your home for the first time is hard for anyone. No longer would I have the comfort of the house in which I was raised for 16 years, the backyard in which my father pitched baseballs to me and in which I chipped golf balls, the neighborhood in which my friends and I roamed looking for mischief, the creek behind the house in which I fished and looked for snakes, the driveway in which I shot thousands of baskets, and the living room in which family time was always spent. These would be just memories now. The difficulty of my move was exacerbated when combined with cancer, chemotherapy, and an uncertain future.

My hometown of Baton Rouge is all of my roots were formed. Knowing every inch of the city, its geography, its culture, its richness, its tailgaiting, its Catholic traditions, its French composition, and of course, its cuisine. Having merely visited other places, I never had to enrich my knowledge of other cities. 1) The water! Uggh. Everywhere else had nasty water . . . hard water that I did not want to drink let alone use when taking a shower. For God's sake, it took a whole bar of soap to get some suds when I visited places in Texas, Tennessee, and Florida; I hoped it would not be the same in Memphis. 2) The food! Can you say bland? Why in the world would someone want to eat food that did not have any taste? Being raised in south Louisiana, I was accustomed to having some flavor and spice in my food; my recollections of vacations were full of tasteless food, or at best, weak attempts at Cajun food by those obviously not trained in the art. 3) LSU sports fans! Any other place in the United States has fans, of course, but they do not compare to the wild, crazy, and often intoxicated individuals who bring their 'A' game to every LSU game; I would not want it any other way. Having visited Austin, TX, Knoxville, TN, and Gainesville, FL, the other Southeastern Conference (SEC) teams try to compete but clearly do not stand a chance. Luckily, I was going to a city that prided itself on their NBA basketball team, a team with which I routed for already.

In addition I would not have easy outlets from the stress of everyday life. Driving to the golf course after school, playing basketball in gym class, and playing video games on the computer or newest gaming system were not options. Just running around the block for several minutes enjoying God's wonders was something that I took for granted; hopefully, I could find other outlets in

Memphis. I did not know much about where my life was headed, but I did know several things:

1) I was very sick

2) Generally, people do not walk away from cancer unscathed

3) I was scared

4) My family would be totally supportive

5) St. Jude's Children Research Hospital was supposed to be THE PLACE to go for cancerous diseases in childhood/adolescent patients

One day, I was told to go to Memphis and the next, I was on my way for 11 weeks. No thought had gone into planning or what it would entail . . . I had to go—no questions asked. What was supposed to be only one week turned into eleven weeks, lasting the entire summer break. After first hearing news of my lengthy stay in Memphis, I felt as though some of my life had been taken from me. I would not be able to associate with my friends during my prime—I was 16 years old and it was the summer. It was time for celebration and fun. My summer would be quite different from any one I had experienced and any one I will ever experience in the future.

Meanwhile, my brother was off on a senior trip—having fun. My sister was beginning her summer—sleeping in. My friends were either golfing everyday or goofing off in some other way. I was jealous that I had to deal with all this crap and not have the opportunities that the others did of enjoying life. Instead of being free to drive around town, I was stuck confined in a one room community-living apartment.

Making contact

Several factors prevented many friends from staying in touch. The greatest contributor was forgetfulness. Most of my friends had multiple circles of friends that could easily occupy their time. Not having one person around was not an 'end of the world' event. What was not there in front of them was forgotten in many respects. Unlike a funeral for someone who dies, someone who develops cancer does not receive a commemorative ceremony. Funerals honor a person's life experiences. Developing cancer, on the other hand, allows people to be forgotten. Those who are ill often have an inability to keep lines of communication open with their friends and family due to physical complications.

Being 380 miles away from me, friends could not easily visit me during my brief stays at St. Jude Children's Research Hospital or my long-term residence at the Ronald McDonald House down the road from the hospital. The phrase 'what you cannot see, you cannot know' played out in my ordeal with cancer. People know that cancer exists, that it is detrimental and even life-threatening, that people lose their hair, and so on; however, until one sees another fighting for his/her life, reality never sets in and the message does not make a personal connection.

Moreover, cancer is intimidating. It is not a fun subject of discussion and thus, it is often verbalized on purpose. Avoiding difficult parts of life and blocking them out is a natural defense mechanism. However, cancerous diseases are becoming diagnosed at higher rates than ever and it is imperative for conversation to emanate regarding how we can better meet the needs of cancer patients. For if we do not provide for those in need, we cannot expect someone to do so for us when we are ill.

"What can I do?" People always asked that question when seeing me during my bout with cancer because appropriate behavior and assistance techniques are not common knowledge for those stricken with or without cancerous diseases. Do I send flowers? Should I visit the person? At the time, I did not have any answers, but through the entire 2 ½ years and through lots of reflection, I have compiled an array of methods by which we can assist these individuals. Many of these issues are contemplated every day by thousands; further recommendations for helping cancer patients are discussed in chapter 23.

One such example involves one of my friends, Elizabeth Marschall. She was a close friend from high school who was also my Physics lab partner. Of course, I always utilized the most refined methods for picking lab partners in high school and college for that matter: 1) select a female, 2) select an attractive female, 3) select an attractive female who was competent, and 4) select an attractive competent female who had a sense of humor. When no candidates fit all of these descriptions, follow the order just mentioned and hope for the best because laboratory classes were heavily involved in mutual experimentation . . . oh yeah.

Where was I? Oh yes, Elizabeth, albeit a close friend, informed me that for awhile she was hesitant to call me in Memphis, TN. Thoughts about "What if I disrupt something going on" or "he might not feel well enough to speak" were some of her concerns. Wow . . . even someone who I knew so well and felt so close to could be scared to call me. Cancer even had that much effect on those who did not even have it themselves. Was it really that powerful or were people just not informed about appropriate practices? Perhaps, the answer includes some of both.

If the circumstances were reversed, it does seem plausible that I would have felt the same way. Being 16 and 17 years old, soon-to-be high school seniors do not have much of a grasp of the real world. Being sheltered in high school is both the greatest and most limiting phases of life; I would not expect anything differently. Having gone through a challenging experience with cancer, I know that instances of reaching out to the ill are greatly desired and appreciated. People just want to feel loved, especially when they are in positions with which they cannot completely control the outcome.

Being a thinker, I thought about various other possibilities why many people had not telephoned me during induction to chemotherapy. In a period where not every high schooler had a mobile cellular phone, I thought perhaps that financial considerations could have factored into not receiving telephone call from many individuals who were my friends. Students in high school were poor, and often depend on their parents for financial assistance, not always having control over long distance phone calls. But when thinking about it some more, I realized that very few parents if any would tell their children that they could not make one phone call to a friend who was just diagnosed with cancer. It would not have cost more than a dollar to pick up the telephone, call my house in Baton Rouge, get my telephone number in Memphis, and make a simple telephone call. It would have taken about one minute and a trace of effort . . . that is all. A simple offering of concern was not too much to ask, or so I thought. Not receiving many calls from friends, I felt as though many people wrote me off completely. Did they think I was going to die? Even still, that should not deter someone from calling; in fact, it might be a greater reason to speak with that person, assuming you care. To this day, my sentiments have not lessened much about the seriousness with which I take the issue. The following is a personal message to those individuals:

Those people who never again associated with me because I was sick- you all can watch from afar, as I continue each day towards achieving something so valuable that you could never understand—making the ongoings of life with cancer public knowledge so as to inform, correct misunderstandings, and change the ways in which these incredible people are treated.

Not everyone fell short, thank God. Those people who visited and called me regularly demonstrated their care and concern for me. One person who has not been mentioned thus far is Jenny Longman. As my first girlfriend, Jenny played a large role to me in my high school years and during my trials of having cancer. We were merely adolescents without too many concerns for what the future would hold.

Being diagnosed with cancer had a life-changing effect on her too. Her first challenge was wrapping her mind around being affiliated with someone who has cancer. Yes, it would be awkward dating someone who was nearly dying. But as we learn in life, shit happens. Once my girlfriend decided that she would stay with me (which should not have been a tough decision but evidently was), a cancer patient, she stayed with me throughout most of the experience. She visited me most weekends (which was a six hour drive), doing whatever she could to bring a smile to my face.

Still, life was difficult no matter who was there with me or what was going on.

The protocol during induction was intense as I received chemotherapy about every other day. Some weeks I even took chemo by mouth (6MP) which caused me to non-stop vomiting all week long. You know it is bad when your abdomen is sore because of the repetitive force of the vomiting. With any and all food spewing from your mouth and nose with speed that could be clocked on a radar gun, patients understand the concept of hell of earth. Pardon the graphic account; it is imperative that the truth be told especially to those who do not want to hear it.

Spending time with my brother, sister, and other friends who came to visit me in Memphis eased the mental stress of being away from home. That week, I did not feel left out; still, they toured the city and participated in various activities while I was at the hospital receiving treatments. Upon arrival, they barely recognized me. When I became ill, I lost some weight from 135 lbs. down to 118 lbs. When they arrived some five weeks later, I weighed 169 lbs. This 30% gain in weight totally changed the way I looked. There were many days when I looked in the mirror, seeing a fat, bald, and sickly looking kid. I was disgusted by what the drugs had done to me. No one deserved this.

Part of the environment at the Ronald McDonald House was the influx of families in and out of the living residence. One day while shooting pool with Seth, one of my buddies there, a girl walked in. Her clothes can be summarized as slacker-style attire. Yet, she was blond, skinny, and had a full onset smile—she entered the room scoping it out, politely walking around while trying to not disrupt our game. About five minutes later, Seth said, "I am going to lie down for awhile." Fatigue was a common symptom of those who were receiving radiation and chemotherapy treatment at the hospital.

His departure left only two people in the room. Samantha introduced herself and stated where she was from and how her sister was the patient. They had just arrived into town and that they would be living at the Ronald McDonald House. She and I played a game or two of pool before I decided to exit the room, saying which room I was in for future reference if she wanted to socialize. Perhaps, I left a good impression with my jovial demeanor. I was sure that I would see her again sometime later.

About 30 minutes later, I had fallen asleep for my routine daily nap. Seth gave me the idea for one when he left an hour before Samantha and I finished playing pool in the game room. Knock, knock, knock. Mom was lying down beside me when we heard the banging on the door. I loved it when Mom lied next to me and held my hand . . . it was one of the most comforting things for me. Going to answer the door, mom asked, "Who is it?" "It's Samantha," said a voice from outside. Mom opened the door (not knowing who this was) and said that I was napping and was not available at the current time. Samantha had already come looking for me after 30 minutes. Hmm?

Around 6:00 p.m., I awoke from a two-hour nap. It felt good doing snow angels in my bed knowing that mom would always straighten it up before bedtime. Once my eyes became acclimated to staying open, I flipped on the television for a bit. I informed my mom that I just met Samantha an hour or two before she knocked on the door. My mom wanted to know what she wanted by knocking on my door, hinting at sexual promiscuity. I chuckled and left it alone. By that time, I was becoming hungry and so we got dressed more suitably and went downstairs to the shared-kitchen area.

While we were cooking breakfast food for dinner that night, Samantha and some of her friends were eating in the dining hall. I stopped by to be polite, saying that I heard she was looking for me. Samantha indicated that her friends were going out that night downtown to some bars and asked if I wanted to attend. I thought that the offer was strange considering I was a cancer patient on chemotherapy who was only 16 years old. In any event, I said that I would not be up for it tonight, declining the offer carefully so as not to blow any future chances with the girl. She was the first person who ever showed interest in my fat-faced, chunky, and sickly looking self with no hair.

After eating my dinner, I returned to our room, where I prepared for bed. Sometimes, I slept as much as possible to minimize my 2 ½ years of pain. I slept a little, but grew restless. This is a common occurrence for chronically ill patients who often sleep during the daytime and then their Circadian rhythm become out of sync. Finally, I got up and went downstairs to get a drink. Walking around for even a couple of minutes sometimes gave me a world of satisfaction. While turning the corner from the entry area to the kitchen, I saw two people enter the building. One person was

Samantha. The other was not someone who I had ever seen nor did he look like he currently resided at the Ronald McDonald House. Although that night, I think he stayed in her room. My question had been answered—Samantha was interested in me as much as she was interested in having her pants filled with some random guy off Beale Street. Classy all the way . . . mom did not seem to be surprised upon hearing the news, nor was I for that matter.

Yet, I was not alone. Most patients had similar types of physical problems in Memphis. Although patients were diagnosed with various types of cancer and blood diseases, there were some medications that were common within most of the treatment protocols. Thus, many of the sick children had the same characteristics as me: sickly in appearance, fat faces, and loss of hair. As strange as I may sound, this in some ways built community relations within the hospital population. Families and patients were no longer treated as different as they might be by normal families and children; together, strong bonds were created between families striving to save the lives of their children.

People from all over the world go to St. Jude to give their children the best opportunity to survive from cancer diagnoses. All socio-economic categories were also represented since St. Jude was willing to pay for all expenditures that one's health insurance refused to pay. Portuguese, Indian, Chinese, Mexican, African, German, and American were just some of the nationalities represented during my first induction stay at the Ronald McDonald House in the summer of 1999. Associating with other people who did not speak the same language was relatively easy when there were universal similarities. Everyone was willing to share their food, supplies, and smiles with each other. This made for having an extended family at the residence.

During the summer after my junior year of high school, several events led up to me making this conclusion. While staying at the Ronald McDonald House in Memphis, I met many other teenagers who also had cancer. I became a close friend of several people, including Courtney, Katie, Kayla, and of course Seth. Our families socialized frequently; however, many times one or more of us felt too ill and not up for socialization. That summer, I was in bed for days on end with spinal headaches, which made me feel like my head was in a vice. Still, I had the natural humanistic urge to communicate and congregate with others. Over time, I stayed in touch with some of the families from that summer; Katie, Kayla, and I were the fortunate ones. Seeing your friends alive one day and dead the next provided me with the perspective that simply being alive was a remarkable privilege that I would no longer take for granted, as I had before being diagnosed with cancer.

Chapter 9:

Coming Home, but not Back to Normal

My stay in Memphis, TN at St. Jude Children's Research Hospital was supposed to be 10 days, or so Dr. Sheila Moore said. There was no plan for 10 days; I think she made up the whole thing for a couple of reasons: 1) So that I would not worry any more than I already was, and 2) With so many unknown factors, it would be impossible to plan for elongated stays. Those 10 days turned into 10 weeks of scheduled appointments, chemotherapy treatments, scans, tests, blood work, surgeries, and agony that actually lasted 11 weeks of continuous residency in Memphis for the completion of the first induction phase of chemotherapy. My blood counts were not high enough during one week to receive treatment and so, an extra week was tacked on to the end to meet the 10-weeks of continuous, hardcore therapy.

Induction was the most challenging experience of my life. Those daily treatments gave me a rude awakening to the real world of sickness, pain, nausea, and many other facets of life I hope to never again experience. My realization of how hard life could be also led me to believe that we should not take one second of healthy life for granted because in an instant, everything can change. Life as I knew it would never be the same; my family and friends also experienced a transformation too.

Bound for Baton Rouge

Once I was released to go home in early September of 1999, I hoped life would get back to normal. For teens, normality began with school. Every weekday from 8:00-3:30 was always occupied with various courses of study. Even though I felt terribly ill, academics were still important. My family and I began to formulate ways in which I could complete high school on time. The task was made more difficult because I would still be receiving weekly regimens of chemotherapy one day per week during the day several miles away from my house at a St. Jude Affiliate Clinic. Those treatments would be given on Friday and thus, Thursdays would be used to conduct lab work so as to determine if my various blood counts were high enough to safely receive chemo that week. Necessary and having priority, somehow I would have to mold my school schedule around those particular hospital visits.

The most difficult factor though was my nausea. I felt absolutely, unequivocally miserable virtually all day long. Not having the stamina or strength to make it through the entire school day was palpable. Although I only needed one credit of English IV to complete the high school required courses, my high school was a magnet school. It was academically-driven and demanded excellence, meaning that high school seniors were required to take a full load of courses. Unlike many other public schools, Baton Rouge Magnet High had standards with which I could not logistically meet during this time of my life.

My father took the initiative, as he always did in life, to setup an appointment with the principal of the school, Mr. Williams. School had already begun about two weeks prior so I was already behind the eightball when arriving back in Baton Rouge. As my father and I entered the principal's office, Mr. Williams pulled out a suggested plan for my senior year of classes. He discussed how I would not have to take a physical education class, and that the staff worked hard on this schedule so my classes would be near one another, limiting my physical exertion and energy expenditure going from one class to another. I looked at my father, giving him a father-son symbol like 'tell him,' and dad began to take control of the situation.

When things work out in life, life is grand. When they do not go your way, life does not have the same bright light to it. But when your dad takes control of a situation just like you had planned, it cannot get any better. My father explained to Mr. Williams that taking all of those classes was not going to happen, referring to my struggles with nausea, vomiting, weakness, and pain. He reiterated to Mr. Williams that there was only one required course for graduation and entrance to Louisiana State University; that was going to be the only course I was going to take this year. My father ended the debate with his no nonsense, bold statements.

Although not generally allowed, I was granted special permission to take only one class, English IV. Mysteriously the rules were broken for special circumstances, just like they should have been. After all, I felt too ill to stay at school all day long and walk around campus. Plus, congregating with the school population could easily infect me with airborne viruses with which my body could not fight off. Instead, I would go to English class each day in the morning and directly leave school. The plan to rest after school took precedence over any extracurricular activities that would have normally taken place. After my meeting with the principal, I struggled up the stairs using my forearm crutches to my English class on the third floor. It took me about 15 minutes just to get up the stairs, almost falling twice and having to ask a stranger to help me.

Upon entering Mrs. Wimberly's classroom, my fellow students welcomed me, seemingly with great surprise in their eyes. Either that or they did not know what to think of me looking totally different physically, using forearm crutches, not having hair, and starting class two weeks into the academic year. The teacher asked that I give a brief update on my status before she continued on with the lesson. While sitting in class, I felt like everyone was staring at me; perhaps, because they really were. Soon, it also dawned on me that just walking up the three flights of stairs made me nauseous. Not only that, but I was not accustomed to paying attention for long periods of time. Even in just 11 weeks of chemotherapy, my concentration and focal abilities were sufficiently lacking. I was used to lying down as well, and even sitting up in the chair for slightly longer than an hour was a difficult task to complete.

Going into English class 20 minutes late on a day that was two weeks into school was exhausting. When class finally ended in what seemed like four hours, I had to leave. Leaving was no walk in the park though. Trying to walk up and down three flights of stairs with hundreds of high schoolers hurrying to their next class was a disaster waiting to happen. That was the most frantic act I have ever witnessed in a school setting. After successfully making it down one flight, I almost busted on the next. That is when I waited on the second floor until everyone was in class before continuing down the stairs. There had to be an easier way. There was no elevator in the school, even though seniors always sold elevator passes to freshman on the first day of school. So I considered alternative solutions like hopping down the stairs while putting all of my weight on my shoulders and arms. That seemed like it would hurt and possibly throw out one of my shoulders. Then, I considered sitting on the stairs and inching down them one at a time. That possibly would not only dirty my pants but also be demeaning. The last possible way that I could conceive would be to slide down the rail slowly until reaching the bottom and have someone carry my crutches down to me. Using this method would allow me to quickly and seamlessly get down the last two flights of stairs without any additional problems. "It should be relatively easy," I thought.

I hopped on the rail, proceeding with caution and carefulness as I began sliding down. Abruptly stopping periodically to slow myself was more awkward than I imagined. Then, I almost slipped backwards over the rail, but somehow managed to stop my fall. Meanwhile, a student was watching and waiting for me at the bottom of the stairwell with my crutches. "You can just leave them there . . . I might be awhile," I said. She seemed very hesitant to leave for fear of me splitting my skull open on the concrete stairs.

Somehow, someway, I made it down those last flights of stairs using the sliding –down-the-rail method. I had expended enough energy contemplating how and proceeding to go down the stairs for an entire day. By the time I crutched over to my car, I was ready to go and never come back. I felt nauseous and ready to puke, so I did right in the parking lot. I did not feel guilty about it either. There was nothing I could have done to avoid it, and I figured that it was some sort of payback for something they must have done to me over the last three years. From school, I drove home contemplating how much of a hassle it was just going to school for one class. What would I do? One thing was clear in my head: there was no way I could keep that up every day. Having arrived back at home, I went straight to my room and fell into bed, threw my crutches down, and went to sleep. This was one thing I knew how to do and being in the comfort of my own bed was greatly appreciated after having spent 11 weeks in Memphis. It was the only place of solace in which I could rely.

When my father arrived home from work, he asked me how the remainder of English class went, since he left the school after the meeting with the principal. I clued him in on the tiredness and nausea that accompanied my classroom experiences. Then, I discussed the dilemma of having English class on the third floor and having to climb three flights of stairs and then descend down them, all on forearm crutches. Dad asked me, "Even if English were on the first floor, could you make it through class on the three days of the week it is held?" I told him that unfortunately I did not think I could do it. Even on a block, 1 ½ hour schedule, attending English class my senior year was too difficult because of the degree of constant nausea I felt each day. On the following day, dad informed Baton Rouge Magnet High School that I could not attend English class on campus anymore.

Instead of going to school several days each week, my father made arrangements with the high school and local district for me to be home-schooled. As much as I looked forward to being the golf team captain, class clown, and socialite, I would not be able to fulfill these duties because of my illness and the pain and nausea with which I was experiencing. Coming back to Baton Rouge was supposed to be 'getting back to normal,' but it turned out to be much more isolation and ongoing difficulties that I did not expect. My expectations were high because I thought this would be my chance to hang out with friends again and reestablish lost connections with my classmates. Yet, it would prove to be complicated without actually attending school. My educational instruction would have to take place at my house during my senior year of high school.

Since I was unable to make it to campus, I was assigned a home school teacher who came by twice a week to teach and tutor me for English IV. Technically, I would remain in Mrs. Wimberly's class but instead of going to school each day, I would complete the same coursework that my fellow classmates were doing in the comfort of my own home. Mr. Chuck, my home school teacher, corresponded with Mrs. Wimberly regularly so that I could remain on track with the others.

The first time that Mr. Chuck and I met, I distinctly recall my father welcoming him into our house as he reeked of cigarette smoke. My father introduced me to Mr. Chuck and explained some of the issues I was having at the time. He seemed very understanding and said that he would work closely with me to ensure that everything was completed. Hailing over 15 years of public school experience and 10 years of home school instruction, Mr. Chuck seemed more than qualified to provide me with instructional support.

Mr. Chuck said that we could start working with some curricular materials beginning the next week. After leaving, my father and I discussed our opinions of Mr. Chuck and what we expected out of the academic school year. My father's opinion has always meant more to me than anyone else's; he has always been reliable and honest and thus, I cared about his opinion enough to ask him what he thought about Mr. Chuck and his background. Without a doubt, we looked at one another and said, "Man, he sure did smell like a smoke stack." Laughing, not at the man, but at the fact that we had the same mindset, my father iterated that he seemed like a kind-hearted personable individual. I concurred and told him that I thought Mr. Chuck was just the right person for my needs. Dad contended that the year would likely still be challenging, but one course should be doable.

That school year, 1999-2000, was a haze in many ways. Being sick for the majority of the time, I do not distinctly recall all of the details and events as they transpired. Mr. Chuck taught me, varying the lengths of his stays and in the number of times he came each week. On the weeks in which my counts were too low to receive chemotherapy, it was agreed upon that he would not come to teach me, for safety reasons of course. To this day, I am unsure of the curriculum for English IV because of the piecemeal fashion it was presented to me and not having the continuity that exists in an in-class setting.

Although my memories of that year of academia are minimal, several parts are quite vivid. I remember going over some information with the man each session and then taking tests on that information the same day. This unorthodox technique was very beneficial in scoring well on the examinations; however, I questioned its effectiveness in having me learn the information. Now

217

that I think about it, that is not entirely true. I did not question anything at the time . . . I was continuing to do what I had done before my tribulations with cancer—finding alternate methods for earning good grades while disregarding the amount of knowledge acquired. In no way am I demeaning the professional abilities of my homeschool teacher, Mr. Chuck. It is my only intention to document how parts of my life played out.

Let's just say that I never read the assigned novels like Beowulf; instead, we jointly took the examinations. Mr. Chuck understood that I could not focus on printed texts for more than a few seconds and so he attempted to mentor me by assisting me with my learning and work production. It was a complex situation because there were requirements that could not be met like reading four novels and writing a seven-page term paper on one of them. I sensed that Mr. Chuck was uneasy about overly assisting me on the tests, but he did it nonetheless. I never asked him for the answers nor expected him to give them to me. He often summarized some of the chapters before we took the tests so as to boost my scores. Both of us felt that this was more appropriate given the situation.

The term paper was the most-weighted portion of my overall grade in English IV. For most students, it took them three to four weeks to complete the assignment. I, on the other hand, did not follow the traditional approach. Beginning the paper on Beowulf consisted of changing the first name on the paper from 'Erich' to 'Evan' and finishing the paper involved modifying the date on the title page of my brother's term paper from the previous year. I guess somebody had to exert all that effort to get the job done . . . and I was ready, like a baseball batter whose team was down one run, to step up to the plate. That was always one advantage to having an older brother who was one grade level higher than me—I utilized the method of using his term papers two out of the three years they were required. So I suppose that my academic dishonesty continued beyond that incident in English class the previous year, but justifiably so.

Although the decision to utilize my brother's work and my teacher's assistance was not always ethical, it was a decision that I do not regret. I was a teenager who needed some extra help at a troubling time. Most of the others in Mrs. Wimberly's class worked so hard on their papers and for that, I felt badly. But that did not

change my feelings about my work completion because I could not
have completed the tasks on my own given the circumstances.
Passing my senior year of high school with straight A's or one A
anyway was a tremendous accomplishment, even though it may not
seem that way to an outsider. Having the opportunity to walk across
the stage at Baton Rouge Magnet High School, or crutch rather, with
my fellow classmates was one of the least expected and most
memorable events of all my high school memories.

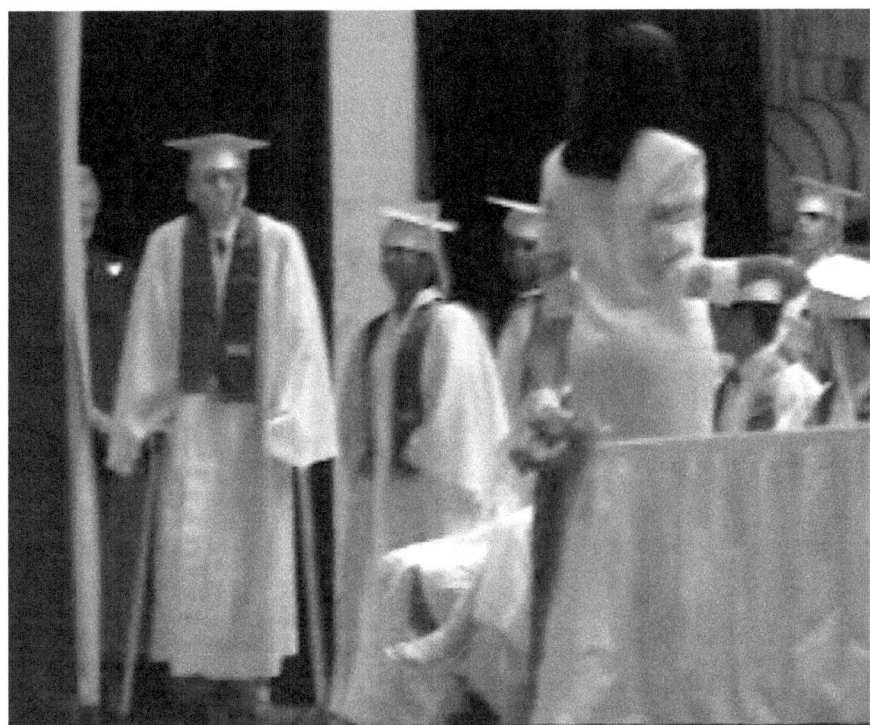

Figure 4. Walking across the stage.

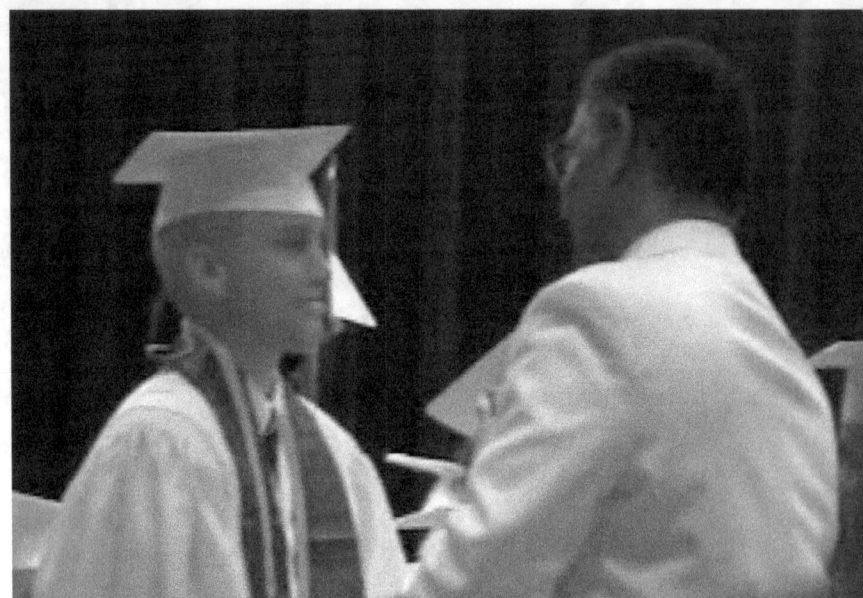

Figure 5. Accepting diploma from Mr. Williams.

Receiving a two minute standing ovation made me feel quite proud of myself too. Perhaps, that would serve as motivation to excel at an all new level.

Having suffered from memory lapses during the senior year of high school, I visited a psychological diagnostic testing facility in Baton Rouge, LA. Several tests were issued to me over two hours before I schedule a follow-up appointment. My father left his work office around lunchtime Wednesday, met me at the location, and we proceeded into the facility to find out the results. Going into the consultation, we had open ears and minds. However we shut down very quickly. The testing center employee informed me that my

221

mental aptitude showed that I should consider a vocational path rather than an academic one after high school. "Perhaps you should think of various trade skills that might interest you," he said. My father and I listened to what the man had to say before collecting the summaries on our way out the door.

As soon as we exited the building, my father said, "I don't care what they say. You can do whatever you want. What do they know anyway?" I agreed and we went our different ways, as he returned to his place of work for the remainder of the day. Still the test results invoked skepticism within my fragile mind. I knew that I was having difficulties concentrating and focusing on academic tasks this year, but I thought it was temporary. According to the tests I was not cut out for college. Should I even try going to college, or would I be better off going to school to be a welder, automotive repairman, or something else that might interest me? These options were seriously considered. During these discussions with my father and family members, Dad stated the he could get me a job at ExxonMobil, where he worked. He said the pay would be good, but it would involve doing shift work for years. The toll on my body that shift-work would cause was not something that I wanted to add to my existing bodily struggles. Eventually I ruled out working at a chemical plant, as well as training in a vocational school too. I was going to college and not just any run of the mill one; I would attend Louisiana State University—the school with which everyone in Baton Rouge longed to attend, the one with which both of my parents graduated, and the one my brother had started one year ago. Any doubts cast on my abilities were ignored for I knew that I was stronger, smarter, and more driven than could be measured on aptitude tests.

Meanwhile, my demeanor was being beaten by the constant ambushing of chemotherapy drips. Just when my body was beginning to get over one week's worth of evil liquid, I was going to do blood work for the next day's treatment. Life was like a non-stop butcher shop, where I was the meat and becoming tortured and eventually destroyed were inevitable. Feeling badly five to seven days a week was wearing on me physically, mentally, and spiritually. After getting chemo, I would be wheelchaired out to my car and then drive home to put myself into a self-induced coma, otherwise known as sleep. However, driving home and simultaneously throwing up did not always go hand-in-hand. After pulling up on a median and puking my guts out one day, I came to the conclusion that I needed assistance going to the hospital each week.

Yet, being the person I am, I was hesitant to ask for assistance. Not certain whether I get the stubbornness from my German, Italian, English, or French heritage (likely the Italian), but my persona beckons me to figure things out for myself and do them myself. I always felt that I was plenty capable of doing whatever needed to be done, so I rarely asked for assistance. Nevertheless, I consulted my father about whom I could ask to take me each Friday. After some thought, he suggested that my grandfather on my mother's side could be a suitable candidate because he had retired several years back. "Seems like a good idea to me," I said. Later that day, I ran the idea by my mother before calling my Paw Paw. She concurred that it seemed like a plausible fit. Upon asking my grandfather if he would be able to help with this matter, he agreed without a second thought, and from that moment, he began taking me to my weekly visits to the St. Jude Affiliate Clinic only three miles from my home in Baton Rouge. Having someone there for me allowed me to focus on my health concerns, which was greatly

needed and will always be remembered.

Chapter 10:

Re-induction

The re-induction phase of my treatment occurred six months into treatment. From November to the end of December of 1999, I lived in Memphis for my second and final extended stay. My family and I planned the accompaniment arrangements in advance so it was much less hectic. Although I was not looking forward to being away again, I had realistic expectations by that time and had already mastered the art of pain masking with games like 'going to my happy place' or 'staying up all night the day before chemotherapy so as to sleep the majority of the following day.'

Family members graciously took turns caring for me during those eight weeks. Although I did not want to return to Memphis, I knew that it was non-negotiable. Plus, I would have various family members there with me so it was my new home away from home. Again, I stayed at the Ronald McDonald House in Memphis, TN. By the time I arrived in November, 1999, they had just completed a renovation of ½ of the facility. It just so happened that I was granted a room in the newer side. I wondered what kinds of improvements could be found in the room. Upon entering the premises, the shared kitchen area looked completely different. It was much more spacious and inviting to families living there as well as their guests. The room, though, is what I really wanted to check out. I opened the door, peered inside, and found a room that looked eerily similar to the ones I stayed in six months ago. There was a television supplied, but the room actually appeared slightly smaller and with different décor. Upon closer examination there were more decorative items like fancy clocks rather than functional ones like cork boards and storage chests. To remedy this problem, my grandfather donated funds for each room in the newly renovated portion of Ronald McDonald House to have a cork board installed. This was yet another example of my family members stepping up to the plate for the cause.

Knowing that I would be in Memphis for approximately eight weeks, I made the necessary arrangements with my homeschool teacher. Two months of time seemed like a long stint without homework and tests, but he did not seem too concerned. He told me to focus on my health and we could make up the missed time with diligence upon my return. I trusted his judgment and did exactly as he suggested.

Unyielding pain. While my father was with me in Memphis, we decided to call it a night one day since we were tired from having sporadic appointments at the hospital. As I lay down to sleep that night, my right knee began to hurt. It was not like an ache or soreness though. Plus, I had not done anything out of the ordinary for it to be hurting, but yet, the pain was intensifying by the second. This was no ordinary, measly pain either. Like a hammer had struck my knee cap, the severity to which my knee hurt was unmatched by any pain I had ever experienced. I screamed for mercy, "AHHHHHH! Dad, uhhhh, it hurts so badly. Please, please call the hospital. Do it . . . hurry! I gotta go now!"

My threshold for pain was extremely high even as a child, but the intensity of my pain in my right knee was intolerable. It was pushing my limits of sanity and as I tried to move positions in bed, propped up my leg on pillows, and tried to walk it out, nothing helped. Rushing downstairs, my dad called the hospital and ran down to get the car. The hospital was right down the road thankfully and we arrived only a few minutes later. Walking with a slight limp, I was not sure if it was damaged and I should take it easy on that leg, or if it did not make any difference. We rode the elevator up to the third floor, the in-patient level. Unlike other hospitals where it takes hours before receiving medical attention, they took me directly into a room, where the patient interview took place.

Of course, the nurse asked me several questions. My interest in what she was saying was null and void. I just wanted the pain to go away. Thinking, "Just go get me what I want" . . . I was not a dope addict or someone who fakes pain for medication. She continued asking me questions related to the pain I was experiencing, asking me to view a pain-scale to determine with what level I associated the pain I was incurring (see Appendix A). Did I really have to see some faces ranging from a smiley face to a frowny face to know that my knee felt like it had exploded? "It was this one," I said, choosing the most frowny faced representation of the choices. "Oh, it must be bad," commented the nurse. I did not know if I was losing my mind, because had not I just informed the woman that it was the worst pain I had ever felt in my life? Was she really that slow or just hard of hearing? Either way, she had better get me some meds and quickly . . . I did not have time to play around with pain-scales and chit chat. I wanted the pain to cease.

After the doctor finally showed up some 40 minutes later, I heard him suggest that I be given intravenous morphine. Immediately, I projected my voice in their direction saying, "Morphine won't touch me! Please give me some Oxycodone. It is the only thing that works on me." The doctor replied saying that they would try 10mg of morphine first and see what happens. I was going mad the whole time, hurting and unable to do anything about the intensity of the pain. But what could I do except bitch and complain?

Needless to say the pain did not subside after the first dose of morphine, nor the second, third, or fourth. Seven hours later, I continued begging for Oxycodone. The overdose of morphine did nothing to numb the pain; at best, it had made me a bit tired. Finally, they agreed to grant my wish; about 30 minutes later, I began to feel relief. And shortly later, my pain had diminished. It was about time! If only they had listened to me first, hours of agonizing discomfort could have been prevented. Inevitably, patients learn and know their bodies better than any doctor or researcher ever could.

It is a most unfortunate and real consequence that many chronically ill and pediatric cancer patients become addicted to type-1 narcotics, requesting medications by name. These instances occur with such veracity that doctors and nurses must use precautionary measures to ensure that children are not embellishing some of their pain to get his/her dope fix. I was never one of these patients for I understood the risks of becoming addicted to drugs, seeing distant relatives and acquaintances become strung out on substances. Still, drug users know that after receiving repetitive doses of narcotics, one has to up the ante to get the same effect. It did not take long before I knew virtually every narcotic by name and which proved effective in relieving my pain.

The knee pain that I possessed emanated from the use of the corticosteroid, Dexamethasone. While its primary function was part of my chemotherapy protocol, its continual use also shut down the blood supply from my bones over time. Blood carries oxygen and when it does not flow well through bones, they become decrepit and eventually die. This is one example of how marvelous and deadly chemotherapy regimens are to the remarkable human body.

Meeting with Dr. Sandlund the following day felt like it was of the utmost importance to figure out what the heck could be done to limit my pain and prevent any future outbursts of intolerable hurting. Sandlund said that the issue was very complex because the steroid, Dexamethasone, was proven to be effective in the treatment of NHL. However, the only way to prevent my pain and my bones from becoming worsened would be to stop the administering of the drug and replacing it with Methotrexate. He said that it is done on rare occasion but that he felt much more comfortable not changing the protocol of drugs. "I cannot guarantee that your bones will get better, but I can say that it is unlikely they will worsen if you stop taking steroids," said Dr. Sandlund. When he sought my counsel, I made my point very clear, "We are stopping steroids today. It's done." My father did not have any objection, at least not verbally. He saw what pain I was in the entire night before and trusted that I could make the best decision.

Although my knee pain finally subsided that night/morning in the hospital, the pain was only a manifestation of the knee bone becoming brittle and weak. Later that week, I took some magnetic resonance images (MRIs) on my knees, hips, and ankles in hopes that the cause of my pain could be known. Those were areas of the body which were most prone to avascular necrosis. St. Jude Children's Research Hospital had and still conducts extensive research in this area of medicine because of both the important and detrimental role steroids play in their regimens.

The orthopedic doctor pulled up his rolling stool and pointed to his screen, showing my mother and me all of the areas in which bone necrosis was present. The scans revealed that my hips and knees had suffered adverse effects from the prolonged use of steroids. Ok? But what did all of this mean? The orthopedic surgeon told me that I would have to use assisted-crutches whenever walking to take the stress off my knees and hips.

Son of a bitch! Why did I need crutches? My knees felt fine at the moment and did not prevent me from walking normally. I could jump up and down if I wanted for God sakes. Crutches were not going to be fun. Soon, a physical therapist came into the room to explain the proper methods for using the crutches. It was not until that very point that I put two and two together. These were no ordinary, underarm crutches. I would be using the crutches in which your arms go into the device for support (see Figure 6).

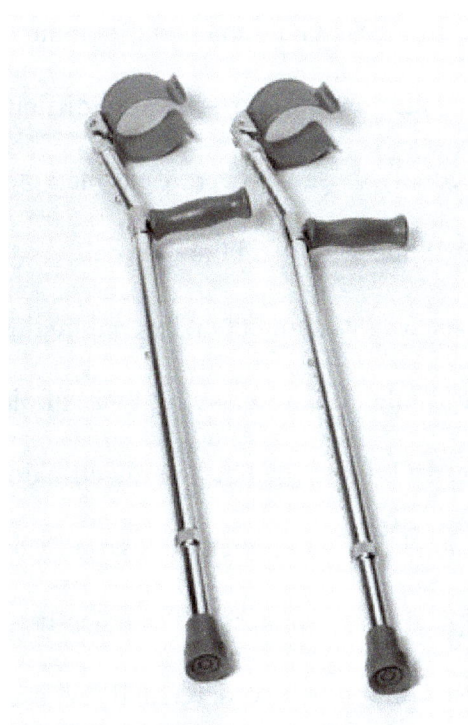

Figure 6. Forearm crutches.

Not only was I bummed about having to use crutches to take the weight off my brittle knees, but I had to use crutches that are often associated with the severely handicapped—another blow to my self-image.

After the physical therapist demonstrated how to walk with them, I realized that it was going to be difficult. I gave it a try and after a couple of minutes, I felt I had the skills necessary to use them, not that I wanted to though. Little did I realize how hard it was becoming accustomed to walking with forearm crutches. Instead of hurting your arm pits, the crutches put a tremendous amount of strain on the wrists and forearms. Plus, certain surfaces were difficult to plant the crutches on, especially those that were wet. I had plenty of time to master the art of walking with them though.

Being scared to ever walk without them, even though my knees did not even hurt me at the time, was weird. I was afraid of doing damage to my knees so I did as the doctor ordered. I do not recall any instances in which I failed to remember to use them. They became part of me, an appendage of some sort. Periodically, I visited with the orthopedic doctor with him who ordered and reviewed MRIs of my knees. Each time, the images looked similar to the previous ones, showing deterioration in those areas. I began to think that I would be on the crutches forever because I was still receiving chemotherapy and it was unlikely that my bones would regenerate, let alone during that time of my life.

Nine months later and still being on the crutches, I spoke to a new and upcoming orthopedic surgeon, Dr. Kevin Neil, who had replaced my previous doctor as the head of the orthopedic section at the hospital. He was heavily involved with joint replacements for patients and seemed like he was of a new breed of physicians.

During my initial visit with Dr. Neil, he said that there was nothing that I could do to prevent my knees and hips from becoming injured. "Well," I thought, "that is strange." Are you telling me that using these crutches was not helping my cause? Dr. Neil said without hesitation that I should not be using the crutches. Allowing your bones to move as normal would actually promote blood flow and most likely keep them in better condition than never having to use them. "Worst case scenario," he said was "if they ever broke completely, they could be replaced. I do a handful of these every week. No big deal." Continuing to open my mind to a new train of thought, he expressed his view that instead of living my life over-cautiously, I should be living as any other teenager—remaining active, exercising, and going places that I wanted. "You mean to tell me that I was on crutches for nine months of my life and I did not even have to," I posited. He carefully responded that he and the previous doctor had differing philosophies of treating my condition. What a bummer that I had wasted all that time on crutches. I tried to take my first step and fell to the ground. No surprise that my leg muscles had atrophied and needed to be developed again. Even so, whew . . . what a relief it was to walk again.

Before I realized, it was the week of Christmas. I was scheduled to receive my weekly regimen of drugs on December 24, 1999. After speaking with my father who was with me at the time, we conjured that if we could get them to give me my chemotherapy on December 23, we could have the possibility of going home for Christmas. We saw that some of the other families were being allowed to go home; however, they lived within two hours of Memphis, or they were not within the induction/re-induction portions of their treatment plan. Nevertheless we decided that it could not hurt to ask. Hesitant as the nurses and Dr. Sandlund were, they agreed to the plan with one condition. My counts had to be high enough to leave and I had to return on December 26. Luckily, everything worked out just as planned and I was able to celebrate Christmas, my favorite time of the year, with my entire family. It was just like old times; except I sat more than usual because of my nausea and of course I had no hair on my head. I enjoyed that miniature two-day break from Memphis . . . it was much needed and deserved.

My grandfather was a huge contributor locally, bringing me to my weekly chemotherapy visits after I realized it was not a safe practice to drive to chemo treatments, drive home, and pull over periodically puking while wanting to curl up in a ball and die. Paw Paw didn't come to Memphis though until my second induction. He stayed with me for two of the eight weeks. It is important to detail this man briefly because I have learned so much from him through our discussions each week. Working from a young age to help support his family, he joined the army and fought in the Korean War. He lived as head of the household, Italian man, who worked his tail off to give his family what they needed. He was a no nonsense kind of man who was sometimes hard around the edges. However, just as developing cancer affected my immediate family, so did it to my grandfather. Paw Paw was there for me and mentored me through everything from politics to personal issues. His 60 years of maturity and life experiences provided a bountiful supply of guidance for which I am truly grateful. I looked forward to those chats, all the while knowing that another chemotherapy drip was going to tear my soul apart.

One memorable occurrence took place one month after my re-induction phase. Arriving back in Memphis, TN, Paw Paw and I went to have a week's worth of tests, scans, and blood work to

238

determine my current status. The purpose was to determine if the cancer was still in remission; the purpose of re-induction was to blast my body once again with a host of drugs like high-dose Methotrexate. The tests throughout the week seemed like they could have been grouped together within about three days. Sometimes, we waited for hours at each appointment. In hindsight, the doctors were saving other people's lives, so how long is too long to wait? I guess I would have waited forever knowing what I know now.

Finally, we finished with the appointments and we were released to go home. My nurses said that they would update me on some of the final tests that were just run, since they had not been examined by medical professionals at that point. Just as we were leaving Memphis in February 2000, a blizzard from the Midwest swooped into town. Being Louisianians, we were not acclimated to the snowy environment, especially when driving on slick roads. As large, freight trucks zoomed by on Interstate 55, we tried desperately to follow other trucks by keeping our eyes on their back lights to maintain some kind of visibility. The storm was almost completely blinding, causing us to slow down to about 35 miles per hour. All of a sudden, the back of my grandfather's truck began swinging to the left side and sure enough, we slid off the road. Maybe an hour or so outside of Memphis, there we were 50 feet off the road, down an embankment, hoping and praying that the truck would start again and we could gain traction to get back to the road. The snow was not about to stop and we just wanted to be home, safe and sound and in the comfort of our own beds. Turning the ignition, Paw Paw started the truck and slowly crept up the embankment at a 45 degree angle without any problem. As we continued down the interstate, we noticed many vehicles off the road, against trees, and being pulled out of ditches by wreckers. We were lucky to be going 20 miles per hour because we were still moving and alive! The snow finally began to subside as we approached Jackson, Mississippi. That's when my grandfather said what we both were thinking, "Maybe you should call your mother and let her know what happened." His comments made me smile because I was waiting for him to say those exact words. All in all, we arrived home around 2:30 a.m. instead of 10:30 p.m., which is still much better than it could have been had we not been so fortunate.

Chapter 11:

Accumulation of Health Issues

During my induction to chemotherapy, I was unsure which was more difficult: dealing with the drugs pumped into my body intravenously or coping with being scared, uncertain, shocked, depressed, alienated, and angry. Why me? What about all of the people in the world who abuse their bodies through choice? Why would a wholesome 16 year old get cancer when there are a million other people who may have been more deserving? This is how I felt for the first month of my stay in Memphis.

While in bed for what seemed like months at a time, my spirituality was tested to the extreme degree. Why would God punish me in this manner? I felt so bad for so long. No person deserved this, especially me. Nevertheless, I prayed to God every day, asking him to answer my questions. Every aspect of life seemed difficult including the physical, psychological, and spiritual. How would I deal with each of these areas of life which were troubling?

Physical ailments

There were both obvious and non-obvious physical problems that accompanied life during chemotherapy. Pain in all of its shapes

241

and sizes was part of daily life. All the pain sensations including throbbing, piercing, radiating, aching, and burning are known by every cancer patient. The tolerance with which cancer patients develop in dealing with their hurting bodies and their cancer treatment is remarkably high. Thus, families and medical staff pay particular attention when patients discuss their types and levels of pain. Associations can be made as to how to treat the pain based on the complaints of the patient. For example, a sharp pain will often indicate that it is nerved-related and can be treated with specific drugs or exercises. Still other instances of pain are unimaginable and the patient, no matter how young, understands his/her body better than anyone else.

Unusual times call for unusual means. My cancer treatment involved extensive use of intravenous chemotherapy in differing amounts of rotating drugs that included: pills, injections, and infusions which lasted various amounts of time ranging from 30 minutes (short drips) to 24 hours (long drips). Every part of my body was adversely affected from the chemotherapy, including my veins. Veins can become damaged or sclerotic when used repetitively for blood work and as host sites for infusing chemotherapy into the body. In addition, some of the chemotherapy drugs were quite harmful if exposed to tissue and/or skin. Known as vesicants, these drugs can damage tissues if drug extravasation or leakage occurs (compartment syndrome). Thus, doctors stress the need for a more permanent line. Central lines, PICC lines, and portacathes are the most popular lines used by physicians.

Aimed at preventing these potential problems, doctors chose to insert a Peripherally Inserted Central Catheter (PICC) into my arm for the remainder of my induction to chemotherapy. This type of central line is inserted in antecubital region and runs up a vein in the arm and finally into the chest, where it reaches the heart (see Figure 7). This is how chemotherapy is fed to the heart and then out to all parts of the body.

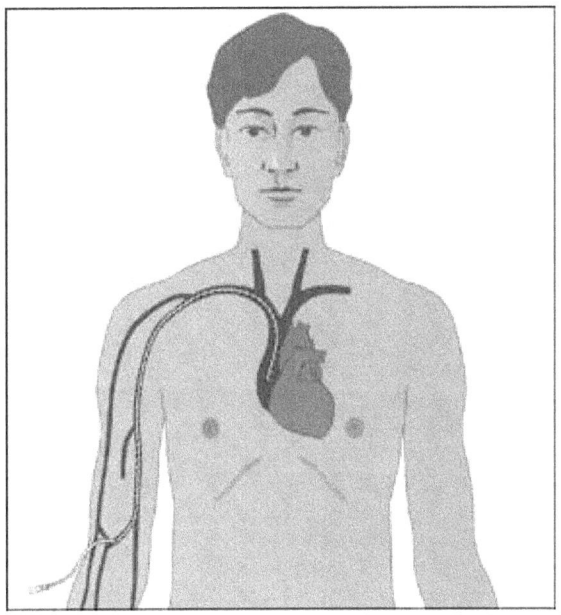

Figure 7. Peripherally Inserted Central Catheter (PICC)

With the PICC line, I had the benefits of the line until they could schedule to have a portacath surgically implanted into my upper pectoral region. Why was an alternate line needed though? The primary reason was that the PICC line and other lines like the

Hickman and Groshong hang outside the body. Concerns about

infection and daily upkeep were of utmost priority for someone who

would be receiving a total of 2 ½ years of chemotherapy. A

portacath is a small chamber implanted into the chest that has an

attached line to the backside that feeds to the heart through a large

vein (see Figure 8). It allows a needle to be inserted into the chamber

or reservoir that is attached just below the

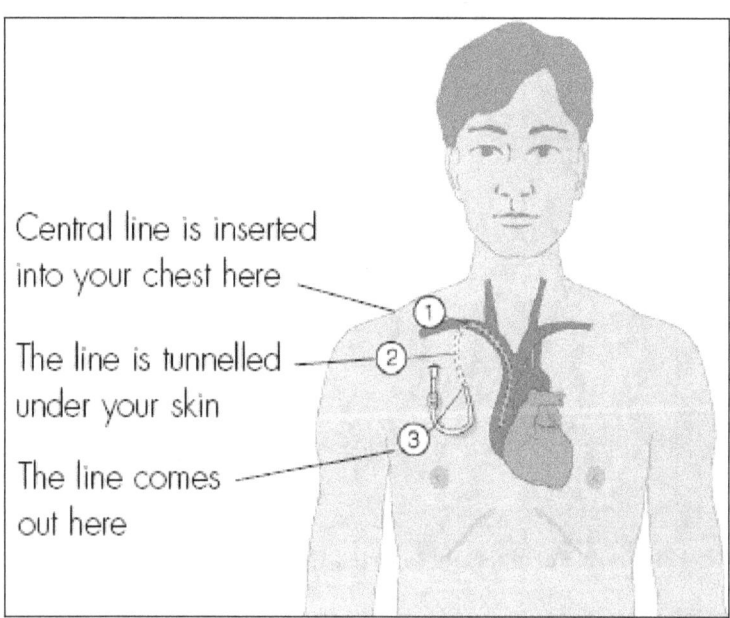

Central line is inserted
into your chest here

The line is tunnelled
under your skin

The line comes
out here

Figure 8. Subcutaneous portacath

surface of the skin (subcutaneous).

Brain damage. Besides having deteriorated bones and a few hardened veins, other parts of my body took a beating from the potent chemotherapy. Treatment called for periodical high doses of Methotrexate (HD-MTX). During induction and re-induction, patients receive high doses within shorter intervals of time to kill any remaining cancer cells. These treatments are so severe that St. Jude will only allow their patients to receive them on site, whereas many of the other treatments can be completed at affiliate clinics throughout the United States. Those days are exacerbated still because patients not only have to endure eight hour treatments of high-dose Methotrexate, but also the accompanied intrathecal chemotherapy that is injected into the spinal column. What an idea— just pump some chemo into your spinal column so that it can flow to your brain. I assumed that these experimental protocols were always carefully crafted by some of the greatest oncologists and researchers, since St. Jude Children's Research Hospital was the greatest pediatric cancer institution in the world, but it did not always make sense to a sick 16-year-old boy.

After seven high-dose treatments of MTX, doctors took a regularly scheduled brain scan. It revealed that HD-MTX had adversely affected my cognition, known as neurotoxicity. Decreases in higher cognitive and neuropsychological functioning were described to me as some of my synapses could no longer connect stored associations and memories as they once could. Less than 10% of my brain usage would be affected according to my neurologist, primarily affecting my short-term memory. Dr. John Sandlund, my primary oncologist, eliminated the remainder of those high doses from my protocol as a result of recognizing my incurred effects up to that point. He felt confident that I had already received an adequate amount of them to have made a positive impression on the fight against the NHL. The extent to which I felt brain damage was uncertain at that point and would not be revealed until I was ready to use my brain as a normal person would each day. All I could focus on was getting well, no time for worrying about anything else . . . anything!

BLAH! The quaint sound of that sweet, sweet serenade of a boy vomiting as his entire body thrusts forward with each burst. Throughout induction and the rest of treatment for that matter, vomiting was a regular and expected occurrence. Most days during those two and one-half years were spent vomiting at least once, sometimes on purpose. I did whatever was necessary to provide even the slightest bit of relief. Often times, substances that resided in the upper gastrointestinal (GI) tract were forced upwards while those in the lower GI tract were forced downwards. The human body is amazing as it attempts to achieve equilibrium.

However, other health concerns surfaced from the excessive heaving. I began to notice that I had feelings of burning in my chest after eating. When inquiring with others, they said I might have heartburn. That was bizarre. Never before did I have any problems eating whatever food I wanted. Maybe I just had a bad day and it would diminish later that night and I would be fine by tomorrow. Positive thinking was going to solve my problems, I tried to tell myself (see Figure x).

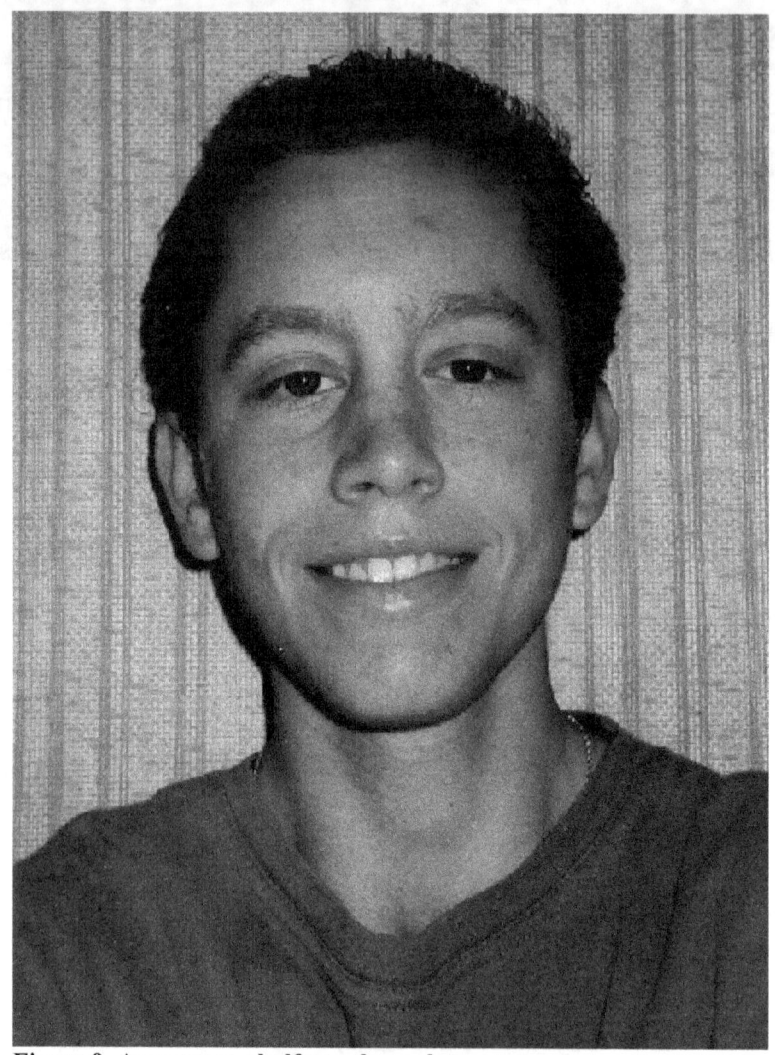

Figure 9. Appearance halfway through treatments.

The next day, Sunday, my mother prepared a nice lunch that featured spaghetti, peas, bread, and my favorite beverage—root beer. I sat down and began devouring the food . . . it was tasty. "Mhhh," I remember telling my mom. "Your spaghetti is the best." Dipping the bread into the spaghetti sauce to give it some more flavor was my next course of action, followed by a big gulp of root beer. "Ahhh" . . . life was good. Unnnhhh . . . I did not feel so well all of a sudden. The burning was back, but this time it was worse. My food was already finished, so I stopping drinking and headed upstairs to sit in bed. My mother was worried. She said, "I bet that acid in the spaghetti did not help it at all . . . I should have known." We would be sure to bring up this issue with Dr. Sandlund tomorrow during our already scheduled weekly appointment.

Upon inspection, my doctor suggested that I receive an endoscopy or upper GI scope so as to determine why I was having these burning sensations because it could be a number of factors that would be treated via different means. Of course, that could not be scheduled for another two weeks, so in the mean time, I was told to take precautionary measures that included eating bland food, no caffeinated beverages, and limit vomiting. LIMIT VOMITING? What? I smiled and said, "OK . . . I'll see what I can do." That was funny, very funny.

Endoscopy. A fairly simple procedure, the endoscopy would consist of the doctor inserting a flexible scope into the mouth down through the esophagus and to the stomach to give a visual for diagnosing and treating a host of conditions like ulcers, intestinal bleeding, esophagitis and heartburn, and gastritis. This 15-30 minute outpatient procedure was completed using anesthesia. Unfortunately, the doctor and nurse who attended to me gave me Demerol, even though I requested that this particular drug not be given to me. In a previous surgery, I realized that Demerol made me feel terrible for hours after surgery, so I always requested it not be issued in future surgeries. Understanding that it is given to control a patient's shaking/reaction, I know there are other meds available and thus, I was disappointed by their decision.

Waking up from the light anesthesia and feeling awful, I began arguing with the nurse about why I felt bad. "It's the anesthesia," she said. So I inquired if anything else was given to me during the procedure. That is when she told me, "Well, we did give you Demerol." What a revelation? No big surprise why I felt terrible. Then, my father chimes in with, "Oh, I apologize for him being disrespectful. He normally isn't like this." Talking about me in third person as if I were not right there in front of him was pissing me off. Then, the nurse and he discussed the causes of my nausea . . . "hello"

I said. "I am right here, fully conscious, and hate it when people do that." Finally, I stopped arguing with them about the nurse issuing me Demerol long enough to learn that my esophageal lining had become worn in several places from repeated exposure to gastric acid, causing me to have heartburn. Vomiting over and over each day had taken a toll on my esophagus and now I would bear the consequence of eating like an 80 year old.

As a result, I had to dramatically change my diet. From fried foods, spicy foods, red sauces, and caffeine—all of which were readily available and very appealing in the South—to non-caffeinated beverages, no seasoning, and no acidic foods. Although my culinary desires would no longer be satisfied, I tried to remember that it was miniscule in comparison to my larger problem. Thus, it was treated as just another mini-obstacle in the race for remission so I shut up and dealt with it.

Fissures. Many of my bodily systems (nervous, circulatory, musculoskeletal, digestive) were indeed affected by the treatments. Like the esophageal issue, I was also faced with other issues from chemotherapy drugs like Etoposide (VP-16). Imagine using the bathroom and only seeing red-colored water in the toilet after standing up. Sounds like fun, huh? Well, I am being facetious of course. Going to the restroom to defecate felt like knives were being pushed out of my body, forming new and more-pronounced tears with each bowel movement. Anal fissures and my back side were as inseparable as peanut butter and jelly. Mouth sores, hair loss, and anemia were yet other side effects from this medication. Throughout this time, my immune system would not readily repair itself because of being suppressed from particular drugs in my treatment. The particular problem of anal fissures was exponentially more difficult as time went on, creating a prolonged source for infection.

As already mentioned, my digestive system did not easily process all foods like those which were spicy or fried and as a result, my stools were not always consistent in nature. Ranging from one extreme to the other, my anus soon became torn and the fissures that emanated did not go away. In fact, they persisted for months; with every bowel movement, blood would flow. Ouucchhh! Every time, the torn flesh would feel like I were a favorite prey of prisoners. Sore and aching, I dreaded each stop at the bathroom. Taking stool softeners and laxatives to regain proper bowel movements did little to prevent the bleeding and pain that became part of daily life.

Fertility. Growing up with an extraordinary father, I was always taught that being a father was an honor and a privilege that I would enjoy one day. A very important part of my future was the prospect of fathering children in the confines of a loving marriage. It has always been dear to me that I be able to father kids like my dad did for me; unfortunately, I was now infertile. Not knowing how to cope with this realization was the toughest part. Sure, people said that I could always adopt a child. But to me, parenthood consisted of raising your own creation from conception. I also dreaded telling any future wife candidates about my inabilities to produce living sperm. More than likely I would be instantly rejected for being less than perfect. To this very day I am still not certain how to resolve this issue as I love children dearly but do not know which course of action makes the most sense when I marry one day.

Sensitivity. Undergoing chemical infusions each week has cumulative effects on one's emotional, physical, and spiritual self. Yes, we can train ourselves to become de-sensitized, or dull. We can even ignore our body's signals; however, those aspects of our lives with which are passionate to us, we actually become over-sensitized to. These areas of my life included friendship, love, sex, drugs, and the promotion of health. I valued my friendships in high school more than academics, and even more than athletic pursuits. That is why it hurt me deeply when many of what I thought were friends abandoned me. Even today when my friendships and relationships do not work out, I am dearly upset. The time investments that I place on friendship cannot be matched by any sum of money.

Love—the only thing more to say about this is that it is the premise of life. To love and to be give love are heartfelt expressions of one's sentiments. Losing a loved one, whether it be a significant other or a family member, causes one to be less than before, for a part of them will never exist again. In our loving relationships we can freely navigate a difficult world with ease. This is why sharing love with cancer patients allows them to live in a much more heavenly like place.

Sex, on the other hand, should be reserved for loving relationships. Otherwise it is a fool's tool at seeking selfish interests or love itself. However it does not work, to which I can readily attest. During my bout with cancer, I used sexual intercourse as an outlet, seeking to alleviate my pain and in the pursuit of touch. The most sought after feeling for me was that of touch. However, it rarely provided any solace and in fact, worsened it more times than not. Why? It is likely that the physical exertion was a contributing factor. However, I was seeking to satisfy my thirst for sexual sensitivity. My selfish interests were likely separate from building relations with my girlfriend. Even though I was in a monogamous relationship with her for nearly three years, I feel as though I used her many times towards this shameful goal.

Health promotion is at the top of my list when it comes to sensitivity. When I see others abusing their bodies with alcohol and drugs, it perturbs me dearly. With time I have become slightly more immune to the rage I would get but the sensitivity is still heightened and will always be. I have felt the negative effects of chemotherapy treatment associated with cancer, but still others act in ways that increase their likelihood of obtaining cancerous diseases. Perhaps my sentiments will mellow more with time but until then, I am glad that all of my thoughts are not broadcast publicly on a regular basis.

Chapter 12:

Conquering Nausea

Ever felt ill? Sure, everyone has felt pain and nausea;

however, nausea associated with cancer treatment is in a category all

to itself. Unless one has undertaken regular chemotherapy

treatments, the level at which one has felt nausea does not compare.

It is not feasible to understand the degree of agony, so instead, I will

focus on explaining how to minimize and control the nausea with

which cancer patients are burdened. Many different techniques exist

aimed at easing the pain that comes with cellular death from

chemotherapy. It is often a trial and error method because of each

human body's unique reaction to medication. Much like radio host,

Michael Savage commented on July 25, 2008 on his nightly

broadcast, developing cancer is likely 1/3 diet-related, 1/3 genetic,

and 1/3 unknown factors. What works best for relief of associated

nausea from chemotherapy treatment is determined by multiple

factors, some of which are not fully understood and often function

on the individual patient level.

The first line of defense against onset nausea is medication.

Various anti-nausea drugs were tried with varying success.

257

Medications range in their approach to relieving the patient from nausea. Various types of drugs include dopamine antagonists, serotonin antagonists, anticholinergics, antihistamines, benzodiazepines, corticosteroids, and cannabinoids. Each specific type of medicine functions to cause reactions in the body so as to achieve the ultimate result—patient satisfaction of a reduction of nausea and vomiting.

The first medicine taken by mouth was a breakthrough drug called Ondansetron, marketed with the name Zofran. Its primary use was for chemotherapy induced nausea and vomiting (CINV). Originally approved by the Federal Drug Administration (FDA) in 1991, it acts as a serotonin 5-HT3 blocker—the first of its kind. These 5-HT3 receptors are found in the chemoreceptor trigger zone and peripherally in the linings of the small intestine (Ramsook, 2002). In 1999, Zofran orally-disintegrating tablets (ODT) were FDA-approved and their use was widespread. That same year, I began taking the medicine, which cost approximately $70 per 8-mg pill. Luckily, those dollars were not coming out of my family's pockets.

Ondansetron was supposed to provide nausea relief to patients undergoing chemotherapy better than previous generations of medications. Indeed, Ondansetron provided some aid. I took the medication the same day of my treatments and days thereafter so long as I remained nauseous. Yet, even with taking the Ondansetron for duration longer than most patients, I remained uncomfortably nauseated the majority of the time. In all, it supplied minimal positive results, so I was ready to try something else.

Instead of using a drug like Ondansetron that is a serotonin antagonist, Dr. Sandlund suggested that I try a histamine H1 receptor antagonist, known as Promethazine. This drug also has qualities of an antihistamine, antiemetic, anticholinergic, and sedative. In theory, it sounds like the perfect drug for those undergoing chemotherapy. I began using it each week instead of the Ondansetron. However, stopping the Ondansetron in order to see if the Promethazine was better proved to be a mistake. Suddenly, I felt even worse than before I began taking this drug. Although Promethazine had once relieved me from nausea from a childhood surgery, it was not effective in relieving CINV . . . at least not as much when compared to Ondansetron.

After realizing that Promethazine did less than Ondansetron to relieve my symptoms, I quickly switched from Promethazine to Granisetron. Beginning with some samples from the doctor, I took the dosage each day in hopes of feeling at least somewhat better. It had already been months since I last felt like a human being; instead, I felt like a subject who was being tortured with cancer, chemotherapy, and mental anguish. Like Ondansetron, Granisetron, marketed as Kytril, acts as a serotonin 5-HT3 receptor antagonist that reduces the activity of the vagus nerve, which activates the vomiting center of the medulla oblongata. Its relatively long life span (4-9 hours/dose) would be especially appropriate for chemotherapy patients, and indeed I did feel somewhat better from taking Kytril. However, the consistency with which I felt relief varied from week to week so I ultimately decided that it did not work as well as the Ondansetron. My search continued for the perfect drug.

Next in line was the Metoclopramide. Having a trade name of Reglan, this medication is a dopamine receptor antagonist— working on the central nervous system (CNS) to provide relief of nausea and vomiting. Its use has been superseded with the advent of drugs like Ondansetron; however, I was desperate so I was willing to try anything at least once. This drug was very different from the others with which I experimented; it had strange effects on the way I felt. Although difficult to describe, Metoclopramide left me with an icky feeling, like there was something in my body that was not quite right. The best example I can use is the feeling you sometimes get hours after a surgery in which anesthesia was used, or the feeling associated with taking narcotics without proper hydration. Metoclopramide was not the silver bullet I was looking for to destroy the bloodthirsty, vampire-like chemotherapy with which I was constantly fighting. My struggles would continue with yet more drugs and alternative therapeutic techniques.

Complain, complain, complain was the name of the game. As I repeatedly griped to my gracious doctor that nothing seemed to be effectively working to aid in nausea relief, my doctor asked me what I thought could help. Wow! A top of the line oncologist at the most reputable children's research hospital in the world asked for my opinion. That was amazing, and simultaneously unexpected. He was supposed to have the answers, not me. I was merely a 17 year old at that point and did not know much of anything in terms of prescribing various types of meds. Without pausing for long, I said, "That's easy. Just put me in a coma for the ~two years left of chemotherapy. Then, wake me up when it is all over." The simple plan did not seem logical in hindsight, but achieving peace was that with which I was desperately searching.

Depression was clearly setting in. My troubled self and sanity were being stripped away each day more and more; hope seemed like a distant memory. It was the opinion of my doctors and parents that my depression and nausea was in some way self-inflicted. Instead of the nausea emanating from the chemotherapy treatments, doctors thought that there was a possibility that as soon as I saw the chemotherapy, I became nauseous from my mental associations with previous drug encounters. There was one truth to this allegation—associating nausea and vomiting with chemotherapy. Other than that, I honestly was disgusted at what they were saying. "It's all in my head, huh," I said. First of all, you would not know because you have never had your veins pumped full of toxic cell-killing agents. Second, if it is all in my head, then why don't you sit in this chair, get hooked up, and take some chemo like a man? Then, we will see what lies in my head and what is actuality.

Having made comments about wanting to be in a coma, doctors tried the next best thing. Benedryl, in addition to Ondansetron, was issued to me each week. The Benedryl is an antihistamine, but it was simply utilized in the sense to make me more likely to sleep for the duration of chemo drips and stays in the hospital clinic. This turned out to be more effective than other treatments and similar to just taking Ondansetron by itself. Eventually, my body began reacting to Benedryl in an alternate fashion. Instead of making me drowsy, it actually pumped me up. Having spoken with several other former Benedryl users, this reaction does not regularly occur, but it does happen in some instances. Again, different bodies react to medications in their own way—reactions are not always predictable. Although the combination approach of taking intravenous Benedryl and Ondansetron by mouth was somewhat effective, my nausea was still sky high. Vomiting several times a day was beginning to be commonplace and my mind continued to be worn down from exhaustion and defeat.

My anxiety for receiving chemotherapy was growing each week; it seemed like an obvious and expected result though. How could one do anything other than be anxious to have those drugs introduced in the body? Dr. Sheila Moore, from Baton Rouge, decided that it was in my best interest to begin taking a new medication, Ativan. It was a benzodiazepine that was primarily used to treat anxiety disorders. Not that I had a disorder, but my anxiety was very real and present each week. Having sedative properties as well, Ativan seemed like an appropriate choice for an adolescent cancer patient like me. I began taking it one-two hours before receiving intravenous treatments. Most of the time, it did seem to make me drowsy, which was a perfectly acceptable side effect for me. I would have taken any medication to sleep more during those years. However, its purpose of relieving anxiety was not recognized. After using it for approximately three months, I stopped taking Ativan for fear of its addictive potential, since it was not functioning effectively in relieving me from my chemotherapy-induced anxiety.

I had had enough. No more games. All of the medicines I tried did not work to my liking. I was prepared to do whatever it took. The type of medicine did not matter to me, as I would have swallowed a rock if it would have provided me with some comfort. Leave it to my mother to suggest alternative drugs for use of pain reduction. Mom said, "I know people in California use marijuana for medical purposes. Why not get some joints to try? Anything is worth a shot." Although marijuana is legal for use in some areas of the country, it was not in Louisiana. Moreover, using illegal drugs went against my moral code of conduct, firmly established throughout my childhood development as a devout Catholic. Never would I smoke dope . . . for I would be just like all those others who I looked down upon for their callous and selfish behavior. Plus, I did not want my body to suffer carcinogenic effects of smoking, so I chose not to pursue smoking pot to alleviate pain and nausea from chemotherapy.

Yet, my mom raised the issue with Dr. Sheila Moore, my local St. Jude oncologist. Her response was not what I expected from medical professional. She said that a synthetic version of THC, a cannabinoid and the common ingredient within marijuana, exists in pill form known as Marinol. "Although we do not commonly prescribe this medication to anyone, let alone minors, we can give it a shot," said Dr. Moore. Continuing to place urgency on the issue, my mother asked if that did not work, could we not just get some street marijuana to try? Dr. Moore hesitated and said, "You can do whatever you think can help Evan feel better. His quality of life is

265

near zero these days, and any improvement would be welcomed wholeheartedly." I debated long and hard over whether to try the $50 per dose of Marinol. Even my religious mentor, dad, purchased the medication and said, "You should try these . . . you are not committing any type of sin by taking prescribed meds for relief from hell on earth." He had a point, so I decided to give the Marinol a chance.

All the hype of disillusioned hippies and thugs on marijuana was not what I expected. In fact, the effects of Marinol on my body were not noticeable at all. At $50 per pill, one would think that there would be some effect on my body and in all likelihood, from a biochemical perspective, there probably were effects. Yet, if it did not provide me with what I was searching for, it would be kicked to the curb. My quest for tranquility was still not satisfied and my use of Marinol lasted only a couple of days—the shortest use of any medication throughout my entire ordeal with cancer. My expectations were not met by Marinol and thereafter, I never had much hope for finding a magic cure to nausea and pain.

Having gone through all the types of meds available to me, I began reflecting on what worked best for me. Undoubtedly,

Ondansetron was the single most effective nausea reliever. Sleeping as much as possible seemed to minimize the amount of pain I suffered, just based on the fact that one is not in pain while unconscious (in most circumstances). My game plan was emerging regarding how to give myself the best chance at minimizing nausea each week during my treatments in the medicine room at the hospital clinic in Baton Rouge. One of my favorite nurses, Di Di, suggested that I receive a triple dosage of intravenous Ondansetron. This would allow me to benefit from its effects for a prolonged period of time. It definitely sounded like a winning idea. In addition, my grandfather said I should try staying up all night long the day before receiving chemotherapy. This would make me naturally sleepy and more likely to sleep throughout the day of chemo. His idea also sounded fantastic. Third, Di Di made a bed in one of the examination rooms with sheets, a comforter, and even a mint on my pillow for my elongated drips. What a sweetheart . . . she gave of herself so much for my sake and this idea was incredible. I was much more comfortable and able to sleep with the lights off in a dark room with no one else around, as opposed to a medicine room with four other patients and their families. Most of the time, someone was eating chicken, playing loud video games, and causing me to be nauseous from the smells, sounds, and lights. Instead, Di Di developed a model scenario for me that has been duplicated for patients ever since at the St. Jude Affiliate Clinic in Baton Rouge, LA. The combination of IV Ondansetron, staying up all night before chemo, and having a comfort sleep zone were the most effective tools in fighting my nausea and vomiting.

Having tried every anti-nausea medication available, my local oncologist was convinced along with some of my family that my feelings of nausea were all in my head. All in my head, are you kidding me? No one has the right to tell a cancer patient that sick feelings from chemotherapy were all mental in nature. I hoped and prayed that none of them would ever have to experience it firsthand and change their ignorant perspectives. That was truly one of the dumbest ideas I had heard.

Instead of medication, Dr. Moore suggested one last thing— that I see a hypnotherapist. "A hypno-what?," I inquired. After, it was explained to me that hypnotherapists allow their patients to use their minds to modify their anxiety and nausea during treatments each week. "Oh, really? Is this person going to make me stand up and cluck like a chicken . . . like you see on television?" I asked. After some sarcastic discussion, I agreed to go to a hypnotherapist— obliging all those who felt I needed a mental adjustment.

I felt hesitant to see a psychotherapist to hypnotize me. What was it going to be like? Besides, I did not believe in all that mumbo-jumbo. Nevertheless, I decided to give it a try. I mean what was the worst that could happen—it would not work and I would be right back where I started. On the other hand, if the hypnotherapist could help me feel less nauseous, it would be a miracle. I guess I had nothing to lose except my dignity, and that was gone a long time ago. It was time to give it a chance once and for all.

Having made an appointment for the next week, I tried not to build up too many expectations. Yet, when I felt so badly each day, it was hard not to hope for the best. I went to the first appointment, which involved little more than the therapist getting to know me and my situation. It was not until the second appointment that she gave me some applicable advice. The hypnotherapist taught me how to relax and visualize my 'happy place.' Mine did not include a midget riding a wooden horse or a half-naked woman pouring me lemonade like in the movie Happy Gilmore; instead, I was playing a round of golf. By visualizing each shot, walking the fairways, and focusing on specific aspects of the round, I was supposed to be less tense and more relieved during my short days at the clinic. Short days consisted of a saline cleansing, a simple push of 5cc's of Methotrexate, and a heparin flush to prevent clotting within the subcutaneous portacathe. This small dose of chemotherapy mildly affected most patients; yet, it made me feel quite sick and thus it seemed like the perfect opportunity to try my relaxation techniques. Each week, I closed my eyes, pictured myself on a particular golf course I had played often, and played a mental round of golf as the nurse injected a yellow substance of displeasure. Sometimes, I began gagging and others I just vomited immediately. Strange feelings, smells, and tastes overtook me. They forced me into puking—the only defensive response my body knew. I sincerely wish that no one has to experience it for oneself, but if you already have, then you know exactly what I mean.

Going home from these visits did not provide much relief either. Sure, I was a bit more comfortable, but how comfortable could one be throwing up all day long for years upon end. Feeling exhausted and only being able to sit around, lounging on the recliner, was so frustrating. It was so miserable not being able to do that which I once took for granted—playing golf, socializing, or going places with family and friends. These were others issues that factored into the mental difficulties that arose from having cancer. Feeling left out was commonplace. How could anyone relate to me if they had not also gone through my experience? Looking back on it, I was naïve. Everyone was going through just as much pain as I was, just in a different manner. Feeling helpless by not knowing how to provide assistance and not being able to help someone feel better were the emotions that friends and family regularly held. Still, I was the one who was depressed every second of the day. To what did I have to look forward, besides more chemotherapy treatments? Even though I had technically been in remission since a few weeks into treatment, the protocol called for two and one-half years worth of chemotherapy to ensure the eradication of the cancer in my body. I questioned whether it was really necessary or was it just their opinion, just like the orthopedic surgeon who told me to use crutches for nine months, only to realize that it was just his opinion.

Chapter 13:

Loneliness

Graduating from high school was an accomplishment that led to a substantial dilemma—now what? Completing the requirements for high school while undergoing chemotherapy was worth noting, but I had higher expectations for myself. College and beyond would prove to be hard to pursue as I continued to feel awful. How could I start college right away? I was barely alive and wishing I weren't. The pain was becoming intolerable and I was sick every day of the week repetitively. Meanwhile, everyone else's lives continued as normal. My brother was doing fairly well in college, living in the dorm room with one of our mutual friends. Not being around him was weird in and of itself; we had always shared a bedroom since the birth of our sister. While in Memphis, I suppose he became accustomed to living life without me around. It surely showed as his concerns were school, college life, and his girlfriend. Rightly so, he had every reason to have different foci than he did while at home during high school. It was just that coming back to Baton Rouge after my first induction phase of chemotherapy lasting 11 weeks took away time that we have spent together. I was looking forward to being back at home, but home was not what it once was. Not only that, but my younger sister was 14 and had her own concerns. No longer would the family exist as it once did. I missed it. I missed being together, socializing, and bonding as a unit. In addition, Monica, my sister, was rebelling against my parents for not receiving the attention which she once had as the baby of the family. It was not fair to her that I receive most of the attention, but in no way was it by choice. That's for sure. Because things were different, now it took everyone some time to adjust to the new scenarios within the extended family structure.

Sitting on the recliner watching stupid daytime television day after day drove me crazy. The only purpose the television played was to keep me company and take my mind away from the world in which I lived. Being by oneself each day adversely affected me in several ways, and many of its signs are still present today. I could not always speak easily after treatments because I hurt so badly that using my voice exerted too much effort and did more trouble than it was worth. Besides, I often became frustrated with people on the telephone as my tolerance levels plummeted. I knew that nothing they could do would bring me any happiness or feelings of being content. Most of the time, I refrained from using the telephone because of those reasons. However, in doing so, I just further isolated myself from those who wanted to show me love in that fashion. My view was that if you didn't have the time to come visit me, then you couldn't possibly care that much. At the same time, I didn't want any visitors either. I did not feel well enough anyway. This cyclical downward spiral of emotions went on for years; some would even say until today. There is no doubt that the psychological effects of chemotherapy and the depression that ensued have tremendously affected many aspects of my life then and now. Even today, I do not use the telephone much because I get easily irritated. Instead, I prefer to interact with people in person; after all, I think that it what life is all about—the relationships we cherish and foster continuously.

Sure, everyone undergoes bouts of depression periodically within their lives. Somehow, this time it felt different though. When it is so hard to imagine feeling well and it is years before you will ever have that chance, it is overwhelming. I had forgotten what it felt like to be healthy or live one day without feeling nauseous. It was true. What was my purpose for living?

Those days from 6-22-99 to 11-17-01 were the longest two and one-half years ever in history, if that is even possible. That time went by on a second to second basis. Reflecting on that period of time seems like it comprised half of my life. When agony is with you each day all day, time is not on your side. The more time you have the longer you feel pain. That is the reasoning for why I longed to be in a coma for the duration of my chemotherapy treatments. What could be better than to not face the daily feelings associated with this battle, continue to receive treatments, and then hopefully wake up years later unscathed? It sure sounded far-fetched, but I was up for anything.

Envisioning a life with harsh treatments, my uncle Kenny envisioned a vacation with which my brother, my cousin (his son), and another Uncle (Keith) could go fishing, canoeing, sailing, and to a baseball game. He made it happen too! I was pumped up about the trip, even though I knew that I would be nauseous for at least part of it. I also hoped that my energy levels could withstand all the fun-filled plans that were arranged (see Figures 10 and 11). The mini-vacation lasted four days but was a release from the harsh reality and monotony of my daily experiences with chemotherapy treatment.

Just like any other vacation, returning home brought with it the depressing reminder of my daily life. I had developed a mean attitude, little or no patience with others, and was tired of dealing with any difficulties associated with other people. Pushing everyone out of my life was the method by which I tried to manage my pain. Thinking that dealing with others was more difficult than it was worth was how my mind tried to make sense of being depressed. Instead, it was merely making me more miserable and lonely than ever before. I eventually drove my girlfriend to leave me. She claimed that I was overly possessive and discourteous to her. Apparently, I had changed. Well

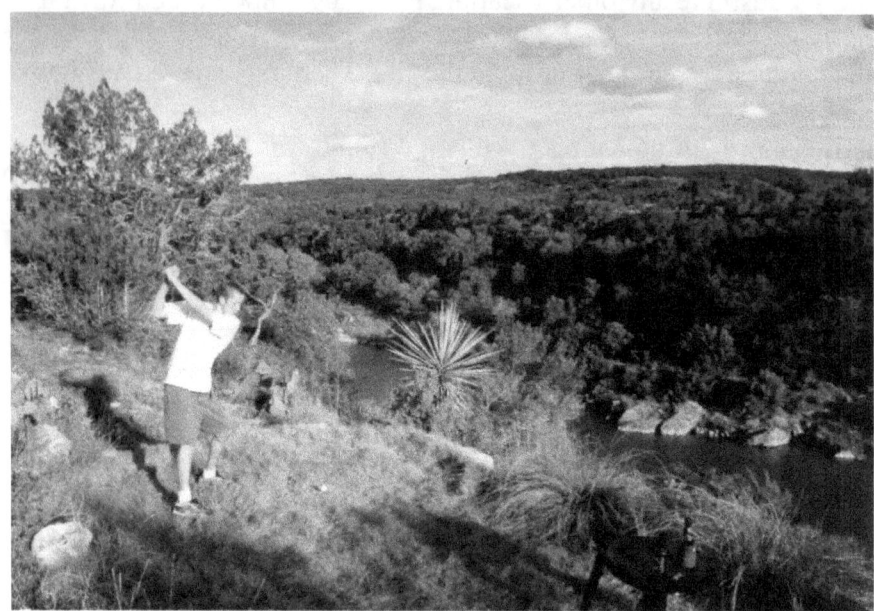

Figure 10. Golf shot over a branch of the Colorado River.

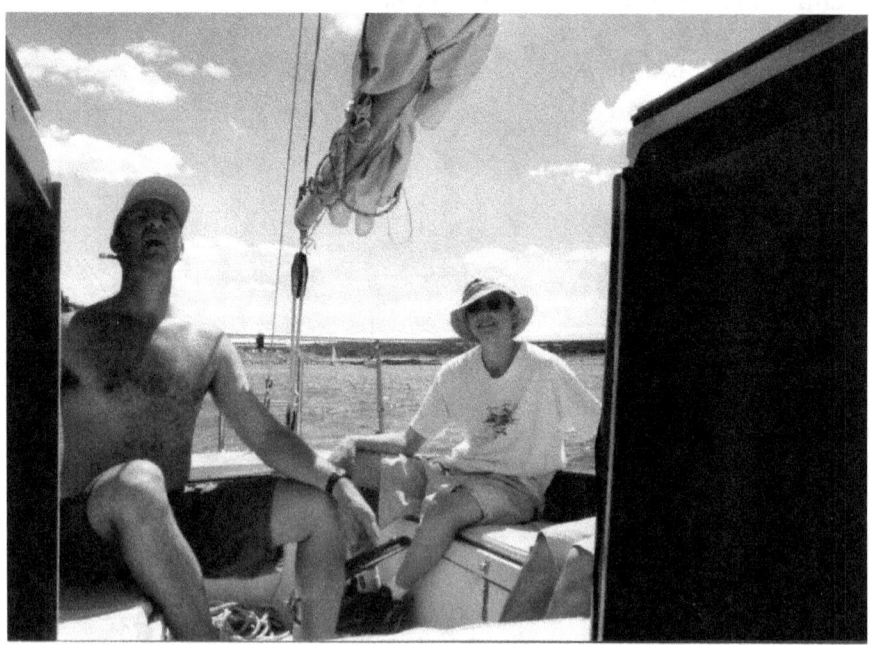

Figure 11. Sailing in Lake Travis, Austin, Texas.

la de freakin dah. I appreciated her earnestness and lack of acceptance of my emotional behavior. On top of that, I had to hear my father say over and over, "Well, maybe if you had not been so mean to her, she would have stayed." I didn't want to hear it. If that is the kind of crap they wanted to discuss, then find someone else to tell. I didn't want to be lectured about my behavior when it was obvious I felt like garbage. Who can be blamed for their behavior when they are being treated in virtually inhumane ways receiving chemotherapy in doses that were supposed to get you as near death as possible week after week. Nevertheless, I was on my own and missed having someone there who I could talk to about my feelings and needs. Shutting everyone out did exactly that.

My weeks were filled with trying to find things to occupy my time. Sometimes, I had to just get up, leave home, and drive. Where would I go? I did not even know my destination many times upon my departure. In a way I was driving to get out of the house. Sitting in a recliner for hours each day was depressing. I left the house in hopes of finding something with which I could relate. It could be that I was seeking to speak with someone, find an interest, or even to try to fit back into society. My adolescent desires to still be a normal, everyday teenager were at the core of my desires. By driving in Baton Rouge with nothing to do, I found myself even more alone than ever. Not only did I have nothing to do, but I had all the time in the world with which to do it. I had no school, relatively speaking. My home school teacher only came by a couple times a week. I did not hold a job at the time either. There were no responsibilities or expectations given to me and my mind and body did not know how to survive this adjustment.

Sometimes, I chose to swing by school around lunchtime for an hour to hang out with some folks on the front lawn as they ate their lunches. Although I sometimes received a welcomed greeting, it was obvious that I was the outsider. When the bell rang, students returned inside the building while I was destined to return to my vehicle before going back home. Other times I would randomly walk into a math class, where my best friend Joey could be found. In those instances it was clear too that he had moved on to establishing friendships with people I did not even know. He had progressed in his life at Baton Rouge Magnet High School, while I was stuck remembering what last year was like. To this very day I still imagine myself being 16 years old, envisioning going to the golf course during physical education class, playing practical jokes, visiting with my friends, and having a typical high school experience. My brother is still 18 years old, my sister is 12 years old, and everything is hunky dory. My development stopped at the end of my junior year in high school and memories of that time will live on forever.

An intellectual void was prevalent during this year of my life when I was only taking one course and being homeschooled. Occupying my time with anything that seemed relatively interesting was my aim when I began to take interest in automotive audio systems. Having newly acquired my father's 1990 Acura Legend when he bought a newer vehicle, it allowed me to pursue these interests. With some money in my bank account from saving virtually every cent I earned, I had some money to play around. Installing a more powerful sound system was at the top of my list. But with the advent of a big sound system came more shenanigans too. I guess I never fully matured in all areas of life. That first car of mine also peaked my interest into the automotive world in general and ever since, I have become fascinated with how mechanical parts work together to function. Perhaps it is the similarity in how machines, like humans, rely upon a multitude of things to produce their greatest output. When one part goes down, nothing is possible.

Just like what the priest had told me.

Chapter 14:

A Renewed Perspective

Through this tragic event in my life, I have developed a perspective that is truly unique. In the past, I felt that giving up seemed like a possible choice. Discontinuing chemotherapy would have allowed me to not feel the pain of those toxic drugs. I would have no longer vomited five times a day or had lines hanging from my arms and chest. Quitting would have relieved me of all the difficulties in my life. I would cease to hurt, feel nauseous, or struggle with mental stress anymore. In a sense, it seemed like quitting chemotherapy would have been a great option. I envisioned my life being back to normal without further chemotherapy. Technically there were no signs of cancer still in my body, but there was a more significant chance of the cancer returning if I stopped the treatment prior to the completion with which St. Jude's studies found to be most effective.

After I spoke with my father about the prospect of quitting my chemotherapy treatments, he called my mother for a sit-down chat. Mom, Dad, and I spoke about the positives and negatives associated with whatever decision I made regarding the possibility of discontinuing chemotherapy. Ultimately, they said that the decision would be mine to make as a 17 year old. However, my father wanted me to speak with the head pastor of our church. His wish was a reasonable request, considering the outcome could have paramount effects. Dad set up the appointment with Father Tom for the following week. Once the appointment was made, I began reflecting on what I really wanted. As a result, I became even more steadfast in my belief that my life was of utter misery and that it was not worth living any more if this was what life stored for me.

While at St. George Catholic Church in Baton Rouge, LA I waited a few minutes in the lobby, as the secretary notified Father Tom of my arrival. He came out, greeting me with a smile and a friendly face. We sat down in some chairs in his office. It was not like I envisioned. I thought he and I would sit at different sides of a desk and argue about the purpose of life. Instead, we were sitting in comfortable chairs discussing how I felt, my relationships with friends and family, and what I wanted from life. He took a holistic approach to looking at my current situation in saying that I had too much ability to throw it all away. The purpose of my existence was not just about me, but for many people. Not only that, but in the future, I could positively affect the lives of thousands of people. Everyone bears a cross in life; this is yours. Quitting chemotherapy would have elevated my chances of dying considerably, and that was a frightening prospect. My father, mother, and local priest changed the way I viewed my purpose in life. I wanted to do more with myself than I could accomplish in just 17 years. How could I have set an example for others to do their best if I had given up? Simply put, I could not. Quitting was no longer an option nor was it ever discussed again. I was focused on what I could do to better the lives of other people. Would I become a doctor and change the world? Would I raise money for research to find cures for cancer? Would I teach children who also struggle during childhood?

It did not matter whether or not I felt excruciating pain for seven days a week, I was grateful for being alive. I had never held such a positive outlook on life. Through this newly-developed viewpoint, I began noticing aspects of my life differently. Instead of feeling like cancer ruined my summer, I realized that I was blessed to spend so much time with many family members and friends. How many other people can say that they spent all summer bonding with their loved ones? Through connecting with them, I gained a better understanding about one of the purposes of my life—to always have positive effects on those around me.

If I could pass high school while receiving chemotherapy treatments, what was stopping me from going to college? I decided not to allow my sickness to prevent me from progressing in my academic career. Soon, I enrolled at Louisiana State University to attend part-time. Concerned family members warned me to not rush into it, but as usual, I did not listen. I had no fear going to school; however, I became terrified after the first day of classes.

After my first class, I went home to review my notes which consisted of three front and back pages of loose-leaf. No matter how many times I read them, I could not remember any of the information. This scared me because I was always a fast learner in school. Unfortunately, some of my high-dose chemotherapy did minor brain damage, affecting my short term memory. How could I pass my collegiate courses, get a job, or provide for myself later in life? All of these questions circled through my head for the next few days. Then, my father taught me another important lesson—in order for my brain to function at its potential, it has to be exercised. I had never thought about it like that. He was basically telling me that my memory would become better and better the more I reviewed the material. Through studying my notes and reading the chapters, I could form more connections between the information. Would it really be that easy?

During the next month, I did exactly as my father suggested. In class, I tape-recorded my professors' lectures and took detailed notes, trying to comprehend the information at the same time. Every day, when I got home from school, I listened to the recorded lectures for hours while reviewing my notes. Through this process, my memory became a sharpened tool. By the time it came to study for the first set of tests, I already knew all of the information in each of my classes. Within a month, 30 pages of notes seemed easy to learn, while three pages of notes previously seemed impossible to grasp. My self-confidence grew to levels higher than ever.

I enrolled in an English service-learning class. To receive credit for this class, I went to Highland Elementary over 30 hours that semester to perform tasks that included observing, assisting, and facilitating learning within a joint third, fourth, and fifth-grade class. By working with these students, I experienced a warm feeling deep within my body. While at Highland, this feeling stayed with me the entire time. I began viewing teaching as a very fulfilling profession. Like Grant Wiggins, a character in Ernest Gaines' (1994) novel, *A Lesson before Dying*, I matured into a purposeful and dedicated teacher through realizing the power of meaningful instruction. This experience significantly influenced my decision to major in elementary education.

My college career has begun on a tough footing but with perseverance, I got the hang of learning, studying, and for once, put forth effort in school. I made a concerted effort to learn as much as possible, for I had a chance to live once again. It was my duty to make the most out of my life. Academics became a priority and in giving my all, I earned a 4.0 cumulative grade point average—a feat that led me to chuckle at the psychological evaluators who said I was not college-bound material. In earning high grades throughout college, I earned several scholarships including those granted by the American Cancer Society (see Figures 12 & 13). All of a sudden I was being commended for my efforts in multiple avenues of life. It was refreshing.

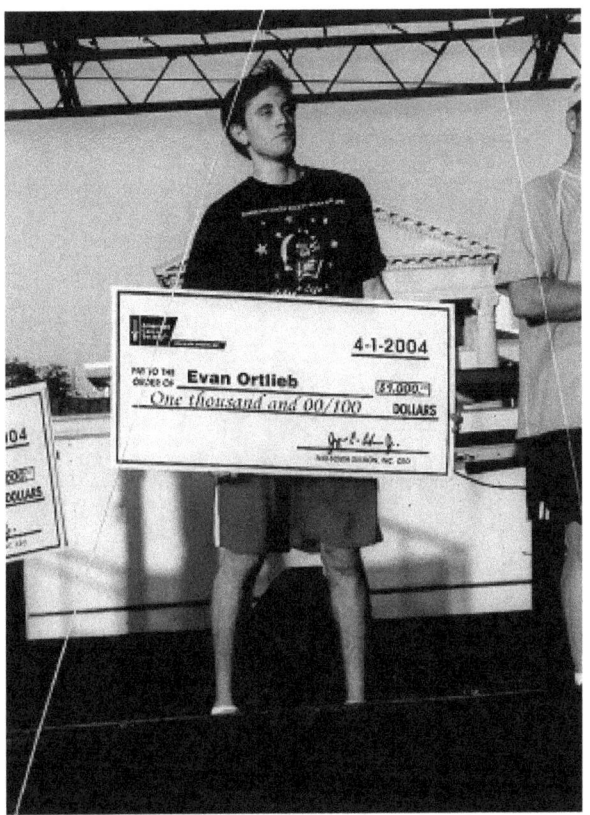

Figure 12. American Cancer Society (ACS) check presentation.

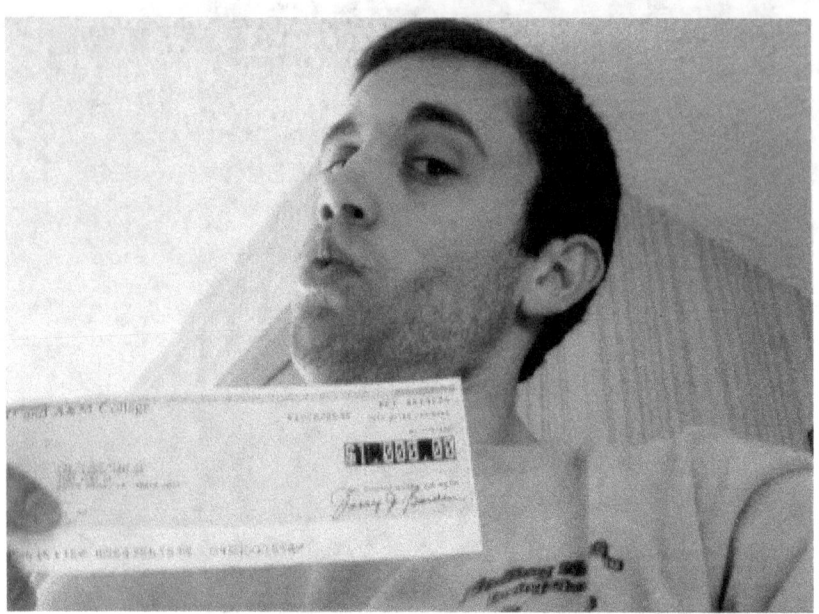

Figure 13. ACS check.

Having realized that my success lied in some ways within myself, I thought that I was capable of accomplishing anything. I no longer expected to fail. Two and a half years after beginning weekly chemotherapy treatments, I finished! Since my cancer was in remission, I would no longer have to experience misery on a daily basis. Now, life seemed easy. At first, I did not know what to do with myself. No longer did I feel sick six days a week. I had enough time to take care of the important aspects of my life, which became more and more evident.

Since then, I dedicated my life to others. Finally, it dawned on me that my purpose was not to die for others like Jesus, but to live for the sake of others. Helping other people would become the focal point of my life; it also brought me more happiness than anything else.

Still each week went by very slowly, dragging and dragging. Once I had a better perspective on life though, it seemed to be a bit easier to deal with all of the hardships that came with my cancer. I developed an alternate attitude to each treatment—I would put my time in and look forward to my after-chemo life. Doing what was necessary was part of any task in life, and I had to look at it that way. If I did what I was supposed to for the good of my body, then hopefully I would be rewarded. After all, I had always been taught that people who do good things in life get rewarded one way or another, whether in this world or the next one. I was finally content with my situation. This had taken over one and one-half years though. Still, I was optimistic about what it would be like cancer-free.

Seeing each day through a newly-developed lens allowed me to live in an entirely new way. Without feelings of depression, life was completely different. I enjoyed being around people and I could understand why I was previously so easily irritated. For instance, when my mother would continually ask, "Do you need something? Can I get something for you?" I didn't blow up, or even get that agitated from those kinds of future instances. I realized that it was love that drove her to offer help and assistance; after all, I should remember that she felt helpless. It was her job as a mother to do what she could to take her child's pain from him; yet, she couldn't put a bandage on it like in the past. She couldn't even comfort me many times because I could not be helped. It was a pain that I had to tolerate. Still, she stayed by my side many days in which I needed someone there. In fact, my entire family helped me on countless occasions, all of which I am extremely grateful for even though I may not have shown my appreciation at the time.

The most memorable aspect of all relationships I had during this ordeal was that between my grandfather and me. He volunteered to take me to my weekly chemotherapy treatments. Not only was this 30 miles away from his house, but he spent sometimes the entire day with me at a hospital. Every Friday, like clockwork he would show up at my door, ready to take me to another week's worth of chemo.

He was there for me, hands down. Never once did he complain or even act as though he were doing something important. He was just filling the gap that needed to be filled. That team work is what allowed for everything to work out.

Being with my grandfather, we grew closer. I never understood certain characteristics about him until I spent lots of time with him one-on-one. We spoke about all sorts of issues ranging from sports to politics to family issues. His views were sometimes different than mine but we always held conversations civilly, never once did they turn into arguments. I learned so much from him during those two years. I would not be nearly as mature and wise as I am today without his mentoring and guidance. He came through when I needed him, just like a true friend; and that he is.

Chapter 15:

After-chemotherapy Life

After some 150 chemotherapy treatments, I reached my final

dose of chemotherapy and I was still alive! On the last day of chemo,

I distinctly remember going to the clinic and preparing myself as

usual for another memorable experience. The night before I stayed

up all night long, not going to sleep in order to hopefully sleep most

of the day of chemo. This was my typical approach to chemo days;

after all, I had tried everything and was a professional by this point. I

knew all the intricacies on how to best prepare oneself for the day of

chemotherapy. Nevertheless, I arrived and the outstanding nurses

had prepared the medicine room just for me. There were balloons,

ribbon, and a cake prepared. I was automatically hesitant to eat the

cake for I knew that it would be upchucked in the near future. Still, it

was the thought that counted, right? I was elated that the time had

finally come. These nurses and staffers had done so much for me

throughout the years (see Figure 14).

Even still, the chemo was calling and I had to face it one

more time. By the way, I decided to eat a small piece of the cake. As

a nurse began giving me the chemotherapy, I started feeling a bit nauseous. At first, I tried to stay calm, but eventually it overcame me. I puked chocolate cake out of my mouth and nose. Burning and only coming out half way, the cake seemed to ruin the entire experience. The nurse felt so bad that she had suggested I eat some of the cake, but I was grateful nonetheless. I sat and smiled as cake remnants and stomach acid filled my nasopharynx. From that point, I foresaw that the world would soon be different once I became well from that treatment.

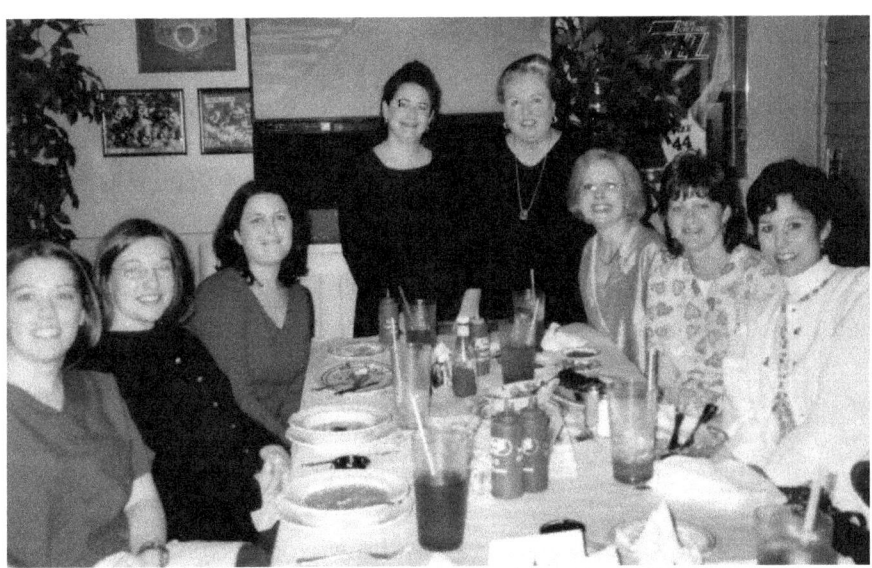

Figure 14. St. Jude Children's Research Hospital – Baton Rouge Affiliate Staff.

About four days later, I began feeling better; yet, my body had become accustomed to being killed by chemotherapy. I did not know how to feel well during after-chemotherapy life (ACT), but two weeks later I realized that I was well from now on. I felt normal! It was impossible . . . I had done it and all that trouble was done with . . . or was it?

Why am I sick?

As great as an aftermath can be, being off chemotherapy was a dream come true. Each day felt so great and so blessed that I had all of my prayers answered. I could not ask for more, not much anyway. Months later, I came down with what I thought was a cold. My throat hurt and I had a slight fever. That got me wondering. What is really just a cold or was it something more? Why was I getting sick? Would it ever go away or was it a sign that cancer was showing its ugly self again? These sentiments of doubt persisted until, well, for years, as I had questions regarding whether or not I would ever get sick again. It is a natural feeling for any cancer patient to have these types of worries; yet, the degree to which one is scared has to do with one's overall optimistic or pessimistic outlook on life.

As I write this memoir, it has been seven years since my last chemotherapy treatment; however, the sometimes faint memories are often remembered during everyday living. For example, when eating deviled eggs at my mother's house one day, I vividly recalled eating deviled eggs one night at the Ronald McDonald House. I was on steroids and had a monstrous appetite. I told my grandmother, who was there along with my mother, "I just thought about deviled eggs." She said, "Oh, well I could make you some tomorrow for lunch." As I looked at my mom before she addressed my grandmother saying, "I think he wants some now." I did not mean to impose my will on my grandmother, but it sure worked. She went down to the mutual kitchen area and began cooking me some deviled eggs. She made six eggs total so that I would have some that night and some would remain for lunch the next day. Well, they didn't last very long. Those 12 halves of stuffed eggs were devoured upon their arrival in front of my face. My grandmother, mother, and I were stunned. What would I have to eat for lunch the next day? To this very day, my grandmother brings up this story, always reminding me of it for its humor, but never to signify her continual dedication to providing for other people. She also had a huge positive impact on my fight with NHL.

Injury prone

Longing to be a teenager once again, I began engaging in physical activities that I could not have while receiving regular chemotherapy treatments. Getting back to golfing seemed like the first activity to try. Normalcy would hopefully be in sight once I was able to do most of the things that I missed. My personality led me to go all out, playing golf as often as time permitted. On one Christmas break from school, my best friend and I played golf nine days in a row. On the fourth day, one of my wrists began hurting me. I just figured that it was sore from becoming re-accustomed to playing the sport again. No big deal, so I kept at it. Well, I could not play on the tenth day because my full throttle style of recreation had caused me to be injured. My left wrist hurt so badly that I could not use it any longer. After going to the doctor, I was told that the inflammation required me to rest my hand for several weeks. Oh well, a small injury like that was not that big of a deal.

Somehow, someway, this injury continued to plague me off and on for four years. Not only did my left wrist "blow out" as I sometimes referred to it, but my right wrist became easily injured as well. For some reason, I had chronic wrist pain and inflammation for years. It became so troublesome that I was unable to use one hand or the other for months upon end, until finally I had enough. I went to one of the best hand and wrist orthopaedic surgeons in Baton Rouge, Rick Ahmad. After months of steroid shots, he finally said that doing a small surgical procedure was the answer. He could easily go in and clean out the inflammation that was giving me agonizing pain. I agreed, and the surgery was completed soon thereafter. Months later, I started rehabilitation, but to no avail. The physical therapy was not helping my wrist; in fact, it was causing more pain and further injury. The surgeon had conducted an improper surgery in that the problem was actually in the capitulate and lunar bones in my hand. The gap between these two bones caused my wrists to hitch, thus inflammation was spreading throughout my wrist area. However, it took a specialist in Memphis to diagnose me. Dr. Rick Ahmad did not even consider this in the nine months of his care. I decided to stick with doctors who knew what they were doing from that point forward. After being told that both my hands would need to be operated on, I knew I was in for a long battle to get my wrists back to proper condition.

Chapter 16:

Role reversal

How would I choose to live life now that I could do whatever I wanted? I was unsure at that point, but I knew that it would be a life full of assisting others just as many had done for me during my challenging times. It wasn't even just about choosing a career, but about how I lived daily. When others needed assistance, I made a dedicated effort to fill that hole. Being there for others is still my goal today. From that time, I dedicated my life to others and in turn, it brought me more happiness than I could have imagined.

My life seemed to be on track from that point. I began taking 18 and 19 hours of school per semester while performing excellently. My family and I were getting along as best as could be expected. Then, I found out that my dad was very ill. He began looking awful in a matter of weeks. Finally, the doctors gave him a message, "If you do not receive a liver transplant soon, you will die." Now the roles were reversed. I was healthy while he was terribly sick. In some respects, it was more difficult to deal with someone else's illness because it seemed like I could not do much to aid him as an outsider.

299

Tick, tock, tick, tock, tick, tock, time went by and my family did not receive any notification that a liver was available. My father looked worse and worse each week. His body began to die right in front of my eyes; his skin became dark-brown with a yellow-like hue. His energy levels declined as he grew anemic. His liver malfunction affected every part of his body including his mind. He became depressed with the possibility of death, just as I did during chemotherapy.

My father was on the liver transplant waiting list in Louisiana for a short time when his dream came true. Dr. Nair made the phone call and said, "You need to drive to Ochsner Hospital immediately because we have a liver for you on the way." As my father panicked while trying to gather his belongings, I stayed calm enough to drive him to the hospital in New Orleans. Approximately 24 hours after receiving the phone call, another liver allowed my father to slowly become healthy once again. From that day, he began to regain his strength and health while never stopping to be the best father imaginable.

My father's liver disease and liver transplant allowed me to be on the other side of the fence. Never before did I truly understand the perspective that all my family members had when I was sick. It seemed just as hard to live life when you know that your father could die at any moment. Another life and death situation reiterated the lesson: Do not take one minute of life for granted. Utilize your time not for monetary gain or notoriety, but for spending time with those who you love. Only then can life be most memorable and meaningful.

Learning how to care for someone afflicted with a grave disease is not easy, nor is having a life-threatening illness oneself. It is in teamwork, however, that any tribulation is possible to resolve. My father served as an incredible mentor to me and my siblings. Even high school and collegiate friends would comment, "Man, your dad is too nice. I wish he was my father." Sorry. There is only one Robert H. Ortlieb, Jr., and I would not trade him for the world. Nevertheless, I live each day now in hopes of closely resembling his lived life experiences because I see how much of a difference he has made in the lives of countless individuals.

Chapter 17:

Life is Grand

Defeating a terrible disease is the largest tangible accomplishment of my life. Going from ordinary teenager to cancer-stricken chemo patient was a difficult adjustment with which had its ups and downs. By no means was I an expert as I navigated through two induction phases as well as weekly treatments. However, I was thankfully associated with St. Jude Children's Research Hospital and trusted in their uncanny research and clinical abilities to get the job done. Torturous as it seemed, the fight was worth it. An eternity of pain cannot compare to the bliss with which life has in store afterwards.

In some ways I have come a long way since my 2.5 year experience with chemotherapy in 1999-2001. I have obtained three degrees from Louisiana State University, including a Doctorate in Curriculum and Instruction with an emphasis in Reading Education. Remaining cancer free has granted me endless possibilities and the allowance to pursue whatever my mind can envision. Currently, I serve as a Full Professor at St. John's University, where I coordinate programs in literacy education. My areas of expertise include the diagnosis and remediation of reading difficulties, reading clinics, and

classroom reading teachers (see Figure 15).

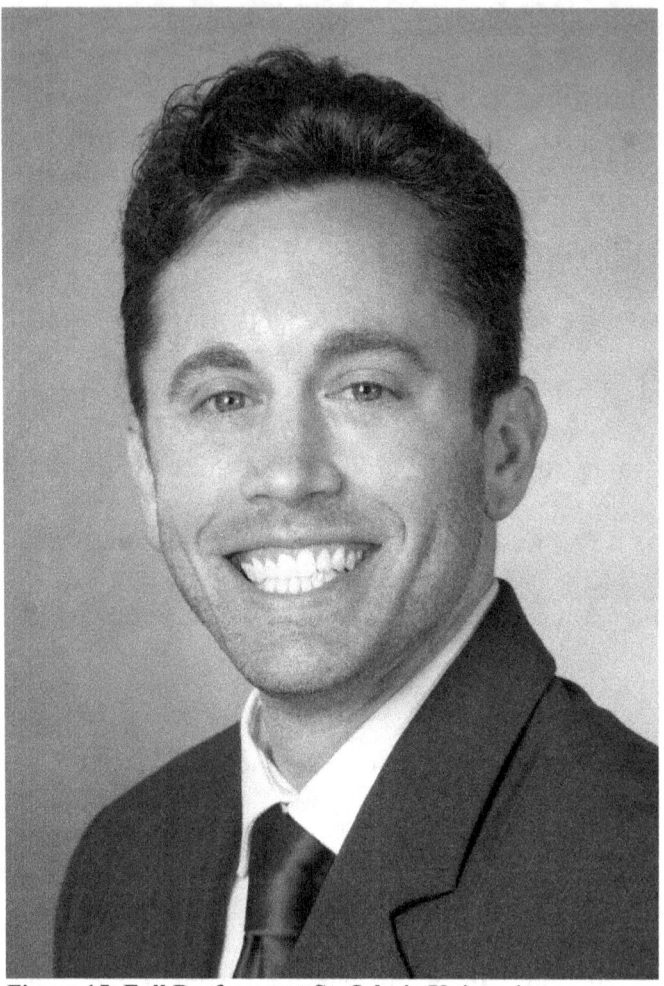

Figure 15. Full Professor at St. John's University.

When one describes life, it is often referred to as being

difficult. Planning, managing time, and allocating time for one's

preferred activities. However I see things a bit differently. I do what

I want. The job I currently have consists of doing acts of research, teaching, and service with which I enjoy. As soon as I no longer enjoy them I will find something different to do. There is no time to complain about life when it is your life and the way in which it is lived is governed by your decisions. In fact I have noticed that I become bored relatively easily these days by having a great deal of time to myself. Thus, I have also begun to pursue items on my list of unaccomplished feats including learning to play guitar, voice lessons, and foreign languages. Navigating life is much trickier when it consists of chosen activities versus scheduled appointment and chemotherapy treatments. It is also quite different not having my family members around me each and every day. The support system that I enjoyed, while pushing some of them away because of my moods, is no longer available in the same form. Instead I must rely upon communicating with them via the telephone—he same device that I once despised. I live 550 miles away from most of my family members who still reside in and around the Baton Rouge, LA area. Being in South Georgia has its perks like allowing me to pursue writing and research efforts more consistently, but there is no replacement for being around one's family. No one is luckier than me for a host of reasons including having the greatest family support system who wish me well and will drop anything to assist me every time it is needed. To show my appreciation for all who have affected my life positively, I have completed and plan to finish several other projects in the near future.

Ventures

In sharing my perspective with other families dealing with cancer, they can gain a positive perspective on what possibilities may come in their future. Positivity is contagious and so, I believe that it can easily spread from one person to hundreds. It gives me fulfillment to meet children undergoing chemotherapy and act as a support system for them. Becoming attached to these children makes me feel whole. As much as cancer patients and their family members need the support of others everywhere, former cancer patients have needs to provide that support. I could not go any duration of time without feeling the desire to be there for these children in some form or fashion. Giving money to St. Jude is an ever-important task and maybe the most important for me to advocate, but it is also imperative that we connect with others while they suffer. There is nothing more tiring than to fight cancer in solitude. Providing any service whether it is through cooking, cleaning, socializing, educating, or advocating is critical to patient success. Medical treatment alone cannot win the battle.

Through my own experiences and observations with other cancer patients, I started a tutoring system several years ago in which college students studying to become teachers would tutor cancer patients in their literacy acquisition. It is in these types of collaborative projects that the importance of meeting the eminent needs of cancer patients becomes known on a broader scale. My collegiate students not only learned valuable teaching skills from firsthand experience, but also developed a life perspective with which was critical for them to be concerned educators of students with special needs.

Writing about the needs of terminally ill and cancerous patients is so desperately needed today. Upon looking at research directed at how cancer patients should be educated, I found only four articles that were written within the last 30 years. In speaking with the educational leadership at St. Jude, Laurie Leigh verified that they customized plans for each and every patient, but utilize the programs in use wherever the patient originally resided. Therefore, if Jane came from Louisville, KY to St. Jude, she would receive tailored instruction/tutoring based almost entirely on the same program that her fellow students in Louisville received. When she finishes with treatment, it would be as though she never left Louisville. This transition is structured to be as seamless as possible. The school re-entry services that St. Jude offers vary from providing relevant videos and written materials to telephone discussions with patients' classroom teachers back home. The school program also "can assist parents by providing information about how to obtain special education services and about federal laws that mandate these services who need them," according to the school program patient information pamphlet.

I understand the benefits of using this protocol; however, there are over one hundred patients living within St. Jude affiliated residencies at any given time. Typically, the school program provides educational services to about 125 patients each year. With only three fully certified teachers, they must rely on a cadre of volunteer teachers and tutors. With ample training and support, it still seems difficult to manage the number of patient needs who have individual circumstances. Designated as a Special Purpose School, the St. Jude School Program is accredited by the Southern Association of Colleges and Schools (SACS). There are two classrooms onsite at St. Jude, one "for kindergarten through sixth grades and another for seventh through 12th grades," according to St. Jude's Promise Magazine (Autumn, 2003). Director of the school program, Laurie Leigh, says "Sometimes all the kids scheduled for the morning show up in the afternoon. That is the essence of this place—patient schedules change and how they feel changes from morning to afternoon." Indeed I completely agree with her statements, but I also hope to add to the existing literature in terms of meeting these students' educational needs while they undergo chemotherapy. Their concerted efforts to allow children and adolescents to continue their normal educational activities and offer "a regular routine, achievable goals, a feeling of control and a sense of normalcy" must be commended. "It is important to create a normal school, because it is what they should be doing. We want to give them hope for the future and let them know that they will get through this," said Laurie Leigh, School Program director. I suspect that patients who utilize these services benefit greatly.

There are still other patients who utilize the homebound approach to continuing their education. During my treatment I took this approach as it seemed that my constant nausea would prevent me from being in the classroom several times a week while at St. Jude during my re-induction. My induction phase occurred during summer so school services were not necessary. However those patients who were enrolled in homebound programs during the school year can have homebound teachers come to the patient's room when they are inpatient at the hospital. International students are also eligible to receive educational services. For those who do not speak English or are not fluent in the language, English as a Second Language teachers from the Memphis area teach these patients at the Target House several times a week, which is located a few miles from the hospital. Most importantly, St. Jude acts to provide advocacy services to patients so they can receive any accommodations necessary, including those in the regular classroom and even related to physical therapy, occupational therapy, and speech therapy.

In essence the School Program at St. Jude is a part of the health care team as it encourages patients to get back to soon as soon as possible for the following reasons:

1) It is a normal childhood activity and increases the child's sense of well-being and reassures the child' sense of being part of the future

2) Maintenance of school social relationships is very important.

3) Missing a lot of school, especially in the early years, can lead to later learning problems.

Thus, their hospital-bound/homebound, school reintegration, and advocacy services provides a complete approach to educating the patient.

Other hospitals throughout the United States have experimented with using technology to virtually integrate patients into their original classrooms. For instance, Georgetown University Hospital partnered with the Leukemia and Lymphoma Society in assisting patients to remain connected with their classes at home via laptop computer with webcam capabilities. Dr. Aziza Shad, MD., Director of Pediatrics at Georgetown University Hospital, states that "you must take care of the whole person. That means taking care of their physical, social, emotional, and psychological needs at the same time" (WTOP, 2009). Staying connected to their classmates, teachers, and school communities is essential to minimize the degree to which cancer patients feel isolated. In the maintaining of these relationships, positive outlooks are much more likely to emanate and prosper. Further utilizing technological innovations will assist many chronically ill patients, not just pediatric cancer patients, develop and hone their academic pursuits and minimize their sense of lost time while they are not able to attend school.

Chapter 18:

Wish-Granting Organizations

My doctors, hospital staff, family members, friends, and strangers alike contributed to my successful victory over non-Hodgkin's lymphoma. With cancer rid of my body, I was free to achieve whatever I could wrap around my mind. But as many who have dealt with cancer and other illnesses, life is not guaranteed. Thus, each day should be seen as a blessing and as an opportunity.

Organizations who donate and provide wishes to children and adolescents with cancer demonstrate this philosophy. Why wait until the child is healed? Today is the day, now is the time. Life is precious and giving sick children opportunities for their dreams to come true should be of central focus. In 1980, the Make-A-Wish Foundation of America was founded to "hope, strength, and joy to children with life-threatening medical conditions," says Williams, president and CEO of the organization. As of 2008, there have been over 167,000 wishes granted. In 2007 alone, there were 13,006 children granted wishes. Today, on average, the Make-A-Wish Foundation grants a wish every 40 minutes. These statistics are mind-boggling and warm felt, having been in a similar situation to those most-deserving youth candidates.

Jordan, a 12 year old, wished to go on a shopping spree, which is a common request for this organization. Instead of the gifts being for him, he wanted to purchase toys and other supplies for homeless children in his hometown of Napa, California. Having read about his story, I felt that everyone needed to know about the wondrous works of this child. For a more expansive list of organizations dedicated to granting wishes to chronically ill children, including childhood cancer patients, see Appendix B. The following is an excerpt from the Make-A-Wish Foundation of America website: www.wish.org

> Twelve-year-old Jordan didn't need a long time to decide on his wish, but his request for a shopping spree from the Greater Bay Area Make-A-Wish Foundation® had a catch. Jordan wanted all the toys, clothes, and other items he purchased to go to homeless children in his community in California.

> Not surprisingly, word of Jordan's wish spread, and two local organizations compiled a "wish list" to help him

identify the items most important to the homeless children. In the weeks leading up to Jordan's shopping spree, retailers and shoppers learned about his altruistic plan and chipped in by making purchases to give him a head start.

With excitement in the air, the time for Jordan's shopping spree arrived. At his first store – Wal-Mart – every manager, associate, and clerk was standing outside to greet him with smiles and tears of joy. Because the big-hearted boy had been featured in a newspaper story, many shoppers recognized Jordan during the day. They offered him words of encouragement and more. Some even gave him money to add to his shopping spree allowance, while others bought items right off the gift registry.

Throughout the day, Jordan found that many of the stores on his list already had carts and bins filled with merchandise bought by shoppers and employees to support his wish. Additionally, every store gave him a discount, a check to supplement his spree, and a special gift just for him!

For part of his experience, Jordan asked to meet the kids who would be benefiting from his kindness. To accomplish this, the Greater Bay Area chapter threw a celebration at a ranch in Napa for Jordan's friends and families, and the families of the homeless children.

The young shopper arrived at the party aboard a fire truck with its sirens blaring. The kids in attendance greeted him with hand-made banners, cheers, applause, and thank-you cards. The fun continued with everyone feasting on Domino's pizza, donated cookies, and Cold Stone Creamery ice cream. The 150 revelers were also entertained with sing-along music, animals, a clown, and face painting.

In addition to the gratitude of the homeless children, Jordan also earned the admiration of the mayor of Napa. During the party, the mayor announced how proud he was of Jordan and presented him with a key to the city! In another highlight, Jordan cried with happiness as he tore open the gift wrapping on his own video camera.

At the end of the day, the families began climbing aboard the trolleys to take them back to their shelters. Jordan gave each kid a hug and a specially-selected present, wrapped that morning by his family and Make-A-Wish®

volunteers. In a fitting end, each child graciously told him "thank you" before boarding the trolley.

The remarkable outcome from Jordan's wish was visible throughout the community; however, acts of generosity do not require visibility for to be appreciated. It is as simple as giving hope to someone; that in itself is the reward. If this sentiment were felt by the majority of the public sphere, cancer patients would benefit greatly. The following accounts from my own experiences demonstrate common retro-perceptions about cancer patients and how these lead to prolonged feelings of anguish. A transformation must emanate, if progress is to occur!

My experiences with wish granting organizations

Foundations that provide hope to sick children are remarkable for a variety of reasons, but dispelling the myth that cancer equates to death is one of the foremost. When the word, CANCER, is uttered or found in print, it is almost always associated with sick individuals who will likely die. In fact, I find myself so bombarded with imagery of elderly people who are placed in the care of hospice workers, sick children with blue marker points on their heads where they will receive radiation, and sickly thin people who look half-dead already. These are images that we see and choose to ignore, turn the channel, or end the conversation; we limit our encounters with uncomfortable subjects. If we thought about these images each day, we would be depressed and in need of mental counseling. Yet, if these individuals, who are just like the rest of us except they happen to be ill at the time, are ignored and shunned by society, their pain will only increase; care and consideration is part of their healing process, and giving anything short of that is doing them a unchristian-like disservice.

As a collegiate professor, part of my job is to make things happen using the power, privilege, and prestige that come with the position. When a deserving, hard-working student needs assistance finding a job, I am always willing to assist. In fact, my former major professor, Earl H. Cheek, and a host of others, including Margaret Stewart and William Doll, Jr., gave me high recommendations which assisted in my landing of my first professorship position. Without these gracious mentors, I would not have the luxury of writing this memoir.

Yet, why are people willing to assist ordinary citizens but not those with cancer? I am contacted exponentially more by friends today than when I was ill years ago. The same goes for many others fighting illnesses such as cancer. This should not be! Using logic, those who are not capable and need the most assistance should receive more than those who need less; however, associating oneself with a less-capable person is sometimes viewed as an eyesore. Hanging around those with less-expensive clothes, older vehicles, dilapidated houses, and blue collar jobs is not 'in.' The Hollywood Scene is what is looked up to, not visiting those in the hospital who are chronically ill.

In addition to desiring popularity, the lack of competency in the field of oncology has led most of society to associate cancer with death. I have heard countless people say that they were ready to die because that is what happens to people when they get cancer. My perspective is slightly different and with more support, a wave of change is possible in terms of altering the public persona—cancer is an illness and with proper treatment can be cured much like any other disease that we obtain during our lifetime.

Those who have experienced cancer firsthand or through those they love do not have this mindset luckily. It is through the perspective, "What can I do?. . . let me help," that teamwork exists.

Of the innumerable methods to help one battling cancer, being a team player is a critical piece of fostering happiness. This statement begs the age-old question: How does one achieve happiness? It starts with living out your aspirations, hopes, and dreams. Children and adolescents dream; meanwhile, adults try not to for fear of not reaching those dreams. Pediatric cancer patients have the same frame of mind; several organizations solely work to turn those dreams into reality, so that they can feel alive and know that anything is possible.

Dreams Come True of Louisiana, Inc. (DCT). This organization was founded in 1982 by seven families from Denham Springs, LA, a city located just east of Baton Rouge, LA, with the intention of providing wishes and fulfilling the dreams of children with life-threatening illnesses. The funding was initially totally contributed by those seven families, but it has since expanded its fundraising efforts to reach children all over the state of Louisiana. An incredible 94% of all donations from individuals, businesses, and fundraising events throughout the year go directly towards cost of dreams for children. Proudly remaining totally encompassed of volunteers, Dreams Come True grants approximately 30-40 wishes each year to qualified recipients—children between the ages of 3 and

21 years old who have a life-threatening illness and reside in the state of Louisiana.

After being introduced to the organization from the same woman who told my family about St. Jude Children's Research Hospital, Pam Bozeman, I began researching who I needed to contact within the organization. One of my childhood friends, Scott Himmel, was involved with the organization in which his uncle was one of the primary fundraising constituents, Max Himmel. He helped me get the ball rolling by telling me who to contact for the 'wish' granting processes. After a simple phone call, I was directed to an individual who was in charge of coordinating the wish-fulfilling efforts, Freddie Smith. She and her husband, Roland, were actually acquaintances of my father and his girlfriend through some casual dance classes they took in Baton Rouge.

Freddie and Roland Smith are two of the most gracious individuals dedicated to supporting efforts to assist cancer patients. After having family members who fought cancer for years on and off again, they felt upset at the world. The perspective is commonplace, but after some time, they realized that their family should be remembered and not forgotten. Carrying on the tradition of helping other cancer patients find happiness, reach goals, and achieve their aspirations was central to their goals in retirement. I could not think of a more fulfilling volunteer opportunity than the one they have; it does not change the fact that their assistance is second to none and has been and will be memorable to all those who benefit from their concerted efforts.

After scheduling a time suitable for all parties, Mrs. Freddie and Mr. Roland arrived to discuss the specifics about making my specific dream come true. Did I want to meet Tiger Woods, the best golfer on the planet? Maybe, I wanted to go to Hawaii for a vacation. Still, I had always wanted to meet some of the Seattle Supersonics professional basketball team players like Shawn Kemp and Gary Payton. These were things that if given the opportunity, I would take full advantage. However, I was too right-brained, too restrictive to pursue those wishes that would just last for a day. I wanted something that had staying power; something that would not be here today and gone tomorrow. That is the reason why I chose a shopping spree as my dream.

Upon meeting with the Smiths, they told me that I would be granted $3000 to spend on almost anything I wanted. Wow! A three followed by three zeros without any decimals was surely a great deal of money; more money than I had probably spent in a lifetime. All of it would have to be used in one outing. These rules and regulations meant that careful planning would be necessary to pull off the best shopping experience of my life. But the greatest question remained—what would I buy with all this money?

I began my overly methodical approach to figuring out what to purchase with this sum of money. It was almost if it was too much money for one who was thrifty and saved his money since birth. Even as a child and an adolescent, the money I accrued from birthday and Christmas presents was stashed away for the future; it was all I knew growing up. My parents always provided what was needed and the extras that I wanted were not bought, purchased as birthday presents, or purchased on rare occasion. Moderation is what made gifts so special; it is what we do not have that remains to be highly desired.

Now, I was in a totally different situation. I had to spend $3000 in one day. Thus, I started conjuring items that could benefit me now and in the future. "Think high-priced items . . . like electronics, technology, and maybe even furniture." I did not have a matching bedroom set of furniture, nor did my family have a matching set of living room furniture. My father's video camera had broken several years before, so it would be beneficial to get one for the family to use with his children who were still living in the house and around town. Also, getting a nice surround sound television system would be awesome because I watched television for hours upon end each day. The only reason being that I could not get up and move around easily being on crutches and feeling nauseous 20-something hours a day. Or should I just purchase items for others to enjoy? Was that against the rules and not even a possibility? I would have to find out.

After my inquiry to the Rolands, they suggested that I get something that I would not ordinarily do for myself. This was the one time in life that was dedicated to giving me something special, and it should be utilized for that exact purpose. Even though I find more happiness in doing for others than for myself, this time I unselfishly took one for the team and chose products to satisfy my desires☺. This realization allowed me to begin the investigation into the specifics of what I was going to buy for myself. After all, this was a once in a lifetime opportunity, so I should make it memorable.

Through mindful reflection and contemplation, I determined that buying several items, including a camcorder and an entertainment center, would be most useful of my conceived ideas. Furniture is something that I really needed to get when moving out of my house, but I was only 17 years old. Having a camcorder would allow me to videotape my friends and family at gatherings, so I could remember them forever. This would carry on the Ortlieb tradition of video documentation. This was a passion that my father had as much as I did; we could share this item and use it whenever the need arose.

Secondly, the entertainment center could serve the needs of everyone who lived in the house and those who came over. Leisure time allows for bonding to occur; having a blasting surround sound system would allow for our house to be the happening spot. Plus, the entertainment center and the camcorder could be taken with me whenever I finished college and moved away. Thus, they would serve my imminent needs and the needs of my future family, for which I envisioned to be with my current girlfriend at the time just like most teenagers do. I have since matured and become realistic.

Now that I decided upon the products that I would purchase, I began calculating how much certain items cost. The following list was the decided upon list of items for which I wanted to buy.

$900   JVC mini-DV camcorder w/ extras

$750   Proscan 32" television

$250   Sony DVD player

$150   JVC 19mm VCR

$550   Kenwood Receiver/Surround Sound Speaker System

$250   Entertainment Center

The shopping spree ($3000) would be completed at Circuit City and Sears. My research began for the best buys for camcorders and entertainment centers, since I could not get off the couch anyway. I figured this would be appropriate, plus I had already been planning since 16 for my future family probably because my father alwayed stressed preparedness and systematic planning towards one's future.

Purchased products included my planned items plus others: a mini-DV JVC camcorder, Proscan 32" television, Sony dvd player, JVC VCR with editing capabilities, Kenwood Receiver and Surround Sound System, Alpine Automotive CD Player with speakers for my brother, and 1 CD: Big Tymers from Circuit City.

Mr. Roland explained the logistics of our purchase and the manager of the store gave me substantial discounts allowing for additional purchases at the store. We finished the shopping spree at Sears where I bought the entertainment center structural housing unit for the television and other electronic equipment.

Having those items fared me well over the years and in fact, I still use many of the products today in my own house. My involvement with Dreams Come True, however, did not cease once my wish was granted. In fact, that was the beginning of a relationship, rather a partnership that mutually benefitted both parties. From the year 2000, I have been actively involved in the fundraising events—speaking to the foundation's supporters, audiences, and patient families in hopes of spreading the word about DCT (see Figures 16, 17, 18, 19, and 20).

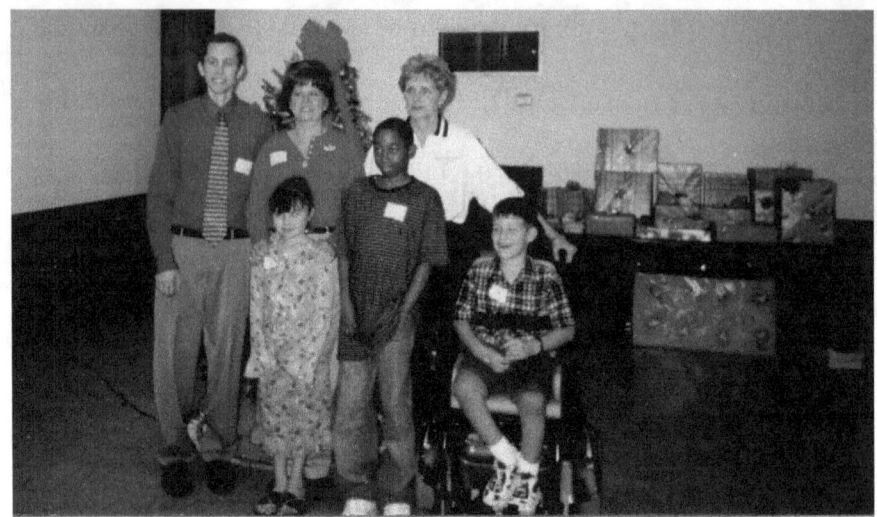

Figure 16. 2001 Christmas gifting to children.

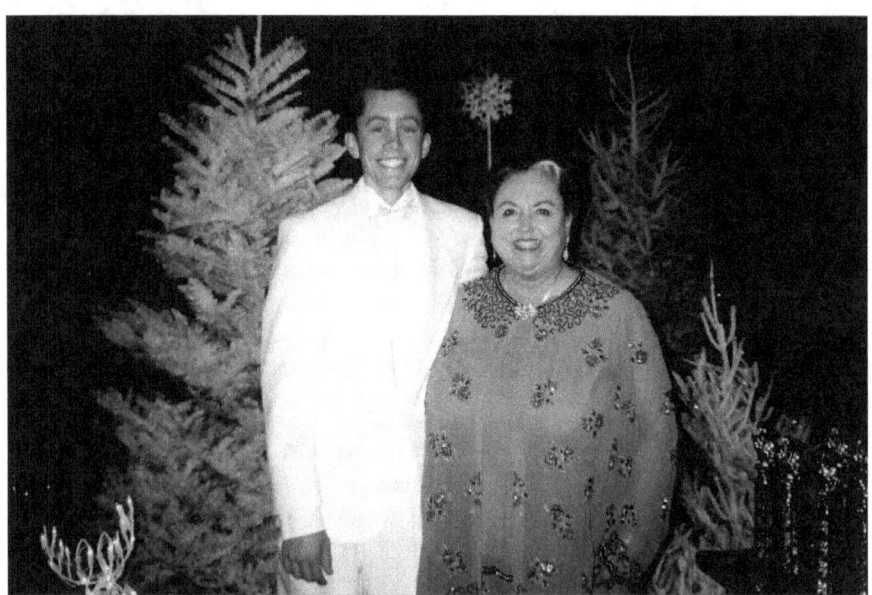

Figure 17. 2002 Christmas Ball.

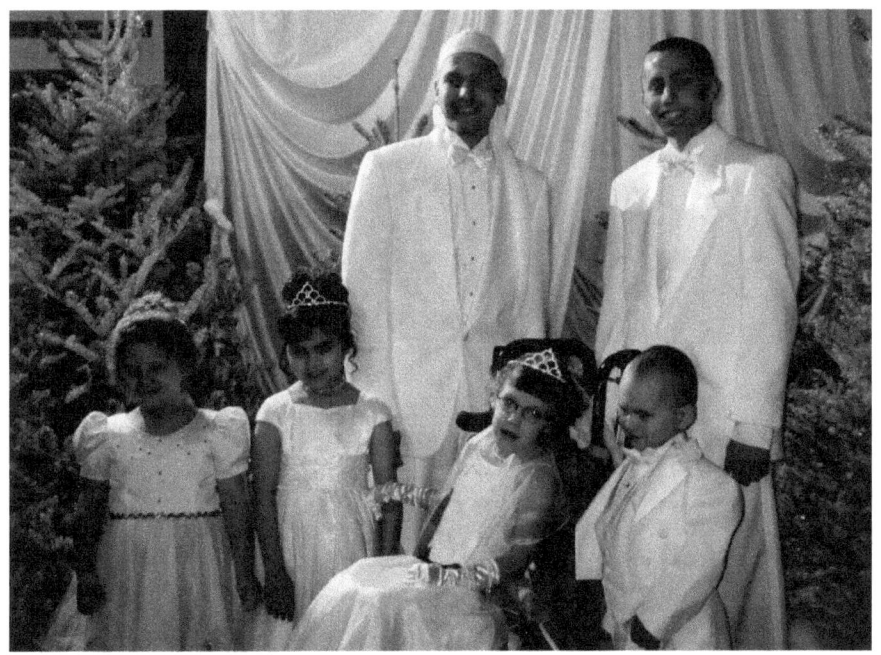

Figure 18. 2002 Christmas Ball (2).

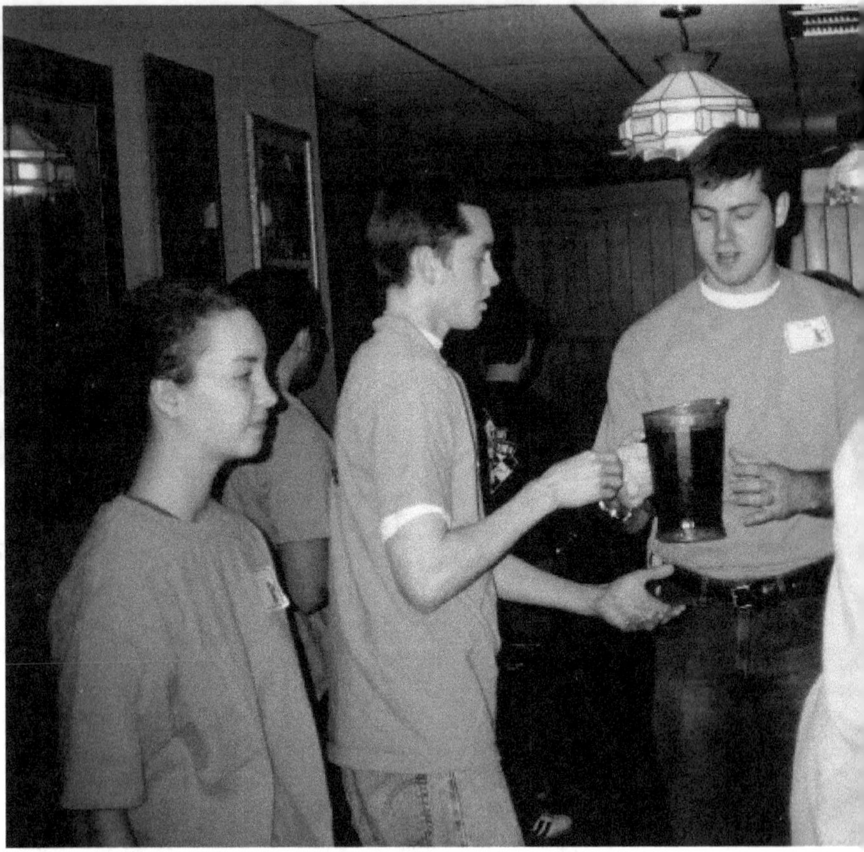

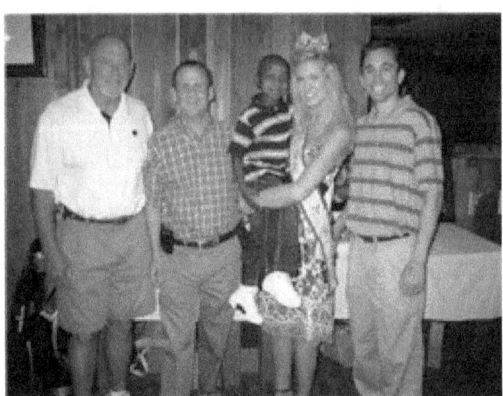

Figure 19. Baton Rouge's Candlelighters rock wall climb.

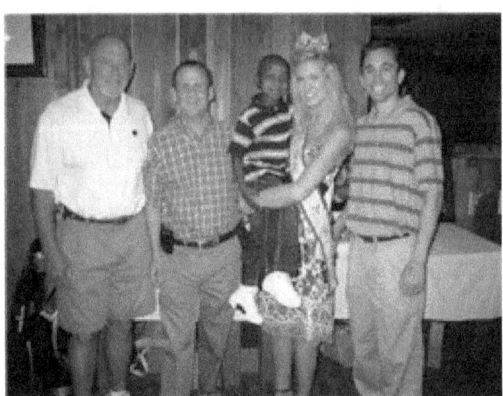

Figure 20. 2007 DCT Golf Tournament Fundraiser.

As a result, I received many accolades that I ignored at the time because my work was and is still far from done. There is so much more to do!

Although it is known that Dreams Come True of Louisiana has assisted in fulfilling children's wishes, the lasting impression and effect on the recipients is not common knowledge. Giving children with chronic illnesses hope not only makes an immediate impact on their lives, but one that spans their lifetime. An attitudinal change results from seeing one of your dreams come true. From what I have seen and lived, attitude accounts for a great deal of one's success. Get a positive one and the rest is history. Just look at the following stories from recipients of DCT granted wishes:

A 17-year-old cancer patient was interviewed in the hospital clinic. His hopes and aspirations of going to college were met with equal feelings of trepidation and fear because he did not have the finances to purchase books, clothes, and other supplies necessary to begin his collegiate career. Dreams Come True granted him a shopping spree for the young man to secure the necessities for him to begin his college career. This scenario of a 17-year-old cancer patient battling for his life is solely focused on the financial impossibilities of beginning college even after obtaining a state-issued scholarship for his tuition (TOPS Program for Louisiana). The burden of cancer is enough for anyone to bear; he should not have to worry about the cost of texts and clothes. Thank God for DCT assisting him to end his tumultuous journey of worrying so he could focus on prosperity.

A 16-year-old boy wanted to see the Chicago Cubs and stay in a luxury hotel, just like in the movie, Field of Dreams with Kevin Costner. After the adolescent was interviewed, the parents spoke with the volunteer privately regarding the severity of the boy's outlook. Prejean, the volunteer from DCT, began making phone calls as she left the hospital clinic. Within two weeks, the boy and his family were visiting with the Chicago Cubs, including hometown product Ryan Theriot. They had a full day there, staying in a 5-star hotel, which was complimentarily provided. In fact, the family said it was their best vacation ever. Unfortunately, it was their last as their son passed away only 3 weeks after returning from Chicago.

The final scenario involves three brothers, all of whom had a life-threatening illness. Interestingly enough, each wanted a drastically different wish: one wanted to see some professional wrestlers in action, one wanted to go to Disney World, and the last wanted to go on a shopping spree. The boys, ages 5, 9, and 10, kept asking Becky Prejean, the volunteer, if she was going with them to Disney World. The ever-energetic boys were sent to Disney World, to a professional wrestling match, and then given a special delivery. A police car, fire truck, and motorcycles arrived at the family's residence to deliver a few of their gifts including a big screen television. The television was especially memorable because the 9-year-old boy is considered legally blind, but can still see when objects are large. The television helped him to see images on the screen, unlike the family's previous small television. In future correspondences, the boys still ask if they can go to Disney again. The volunteer says no but still gets hugs from all of them. Becky Prejean of DCT summed up her experiences of volunteering by saying:

> Things that we take for granted, like refrigerators, living room furniture, bedroom sets, and food are so important to those in need. The expressions on their faces when we walk out of a store with those goods or even their own computer, cell phone, camera, TV, nice clothes, shoes, and jewelry, no

money can replace. They feel so good about themselves!

When I get in my car, that is when I know it is all worth what we do. That is our payment.

Make-A-Wish Foundation. This organization is widely known for its efforts across the entire United States for granting wishes to youth with life-threatening illnesses. However, I was not introduced to the organization until one of my favorite nurses, Di Di, told me about how they work with her patients regularly in granting their wishes. But did I not just have a wish granted from organization-Dreams Come True? Each organization was completely separate; in fact, there were many, many organizations throughout the United States that make children's wishes come true (see Appendix B). I was content though with having been granted my wish; Dreams Come True had done so much for me that would assist me now and into adulthood. Then, while in the hospital clinic on Friday about to receive a dose of chemo, I met a representative from the Make-A-Wish Foundation, who was there to interview another patient. She said that she would schedule an appointment to see me in the near future.

Mhhh . . . did this mean I was about to score a $5000 shopping spree on top of the $3000 one I already received from Dreams Come True? I did not pry into trying to mooch from the Make-A-Wish Foundation; they contacted me, scheduled the appointment, interviewed me, and informed me of when the shopping spree would occur. Wow! This was déjà vu all over again. More stuff to set up my future. Since I had already purchased some items like an entertainment center and video camera, I figured that I would need some furniture in this futuristic place of my residence.

Quickly learning that furniture is not cheap, I made the determination that I would either purchase a bedroom set or a living room set of furniture. My girlfriend and I scoped out all the furniture stores in Baton Rouge, LA to see what types of goods they had, just to get some ideas. Even though I was warned, I was astonished at the high costs associated with furniture bought at reputable furnishing stores. In this instance, however, I did not have to worry about the costs. Now, for the second time in my life, money was not an issue; instead, I could get exactly what I wanted. For the bedroom set, I had my eyes on a sleigh bed set with dark mahogany wood. It sure beat out my current bed without a headboard and footboard, alongside two mismatching dressers with broken drawers and missing handles. The set cost about $4000, which was entirely too expensive, except I was encouraged to spend the entire sum of money that would be granted. So, like in the Disney's Lion King, I lived by the adage—hakuna matata: No worries.

Upon examining all of the various mattresses available, I must have lied on 50 or so before falling in love with one queen mattress and box spring that cost just under $1000. This amount of money was more than the furniture in my entire house was worth. Crazy as it seemed, I was determined to get the best bang for my buck, rather Make-A-Wish Foundation's buck. Still, I was not totally set on bedroom furniture. My father's house might not be able to accommodate the five-piece set of furniture easily into my 12 x 13 room. Therefore, I continued to look around for some pieces of living room furniture and if I found one to my liking, I would just go in that direction instead.

The Sunday newspaper seemed like a good place to start perusing advertisements for living room furniture. The Advocate, Baton Rouge's newspaper, always contained many ads on Sundays for sales on merchandise. Between the newspaper and the yellow pages, I found many stores that specialized in home furnishing besides the ones I had already visited looking for bedroom furniture. I drove to most of them on the next couple of days, since I was still not in school at the time. The businesses varied greatly in quality, price, and selection. One of the problems associated with shopping in general is first having an idea of what you want; without having predetermined that much, it is difficult to find something that you like. Somehow though, I stumbled upon two couches that I thought were perfect. A three-cushion couch and a loveseat were off-white colored and so comfortable. Most couches I had tested either forced me to slouch significantly or they made me sit totally upright. These were different. They had it all, and at only $2000, they would allow me to buy some other items. Even a new mattress would be easily within my price range. I could also get a brand new recliner, which was so critical to my couch-potato endeavors during my sickness. The current recliner that was in my dad's living room was beginning to lean a bit and it would soon need to be replaced anyway. This $5000 shopping spree was now tangible—my list was set. Now, I would wait two weeks until the representative from the Make-A-Wish Foundation would meet my family and me.

One week passed and the rep called me to review the time for the meeting. She asked me several last questions to ensure everything would run smoothly. But it did not! The third question uttered, "You haven't received any other wishes granted by any other organizations, right?" Excuse me! "Actually, I have," I explained. "Dreams Come True of Louisiana granted me a wish several months ago." "Oh," she said. "Then, I should let you know that we do not grant wishes to individuals who have already been wish recipients from us or any other organization. I am so sorry." A minute later the conversation was completed and so were my thoughts of getting a second wish. Lesson learned—your first thoughts on a subject are probably accurate, like how I questioned whether it was proper for me to receive a second wish. Oh well.

Odd wishes. In December of 2001, the Chicago Sun Times' Benjamin Errett reported that earlier in the month, "a terminally ill boy had his dying wish granted in Australia this month" (p. 1). Unlike other wishes like meeting movie stars and going to places like Disneyland, this anonymous 15 year old wanted to experience something with which many teenagers are curious—sex. He wanted to lose his virginity before dying of cancer. Without parental or hospital consent, some of his friends arranged an encounter with a prostitute. In fact, some of the hospital staff wanted to pool together monies to pay for the meeting. Judy Lumby, the executive director of the New South Wales College of Nursing, added:

> I would try my darndest as a nurse to do whatever I could to make sure his wish came true. I just think we are so archaic in the way we treat people in institutions. Certainly, if any of my three daughters were dying, I'd do whatever I could, and I'm sure that you would, too."

According to Errett (2001), "Because of his many years in the hospital, he had no girlfriend or female friends" (p. 1). Whether or not you agree with the actions taken by the boy, his friends, and the prostitute, there is a larger underlying psychological issue at hand. The cancer patient's desire for a sexual encounter was in part due to his conditioning of receiving unpleasant, hurtful instances of touch. Every time he received treatments with nurses, doctors, and others touching him, mental associations were created. However, the need for basic human contact remains with us for life. Thus, children receiving treatment or dying over a long period of time can sometimes develop a condition known as 'skin hunger,' according to Dr. Leeder, Dean of Medicine at the University of Sydney.

In a conversation that emanated from hearing about this story while listening to the radio, my mother commented that she would have paid for me to have sex if that was my wish if I were dying. The man on the radio expressed similar sentiments that he would have raised money to hire a prostitute to service the 15-year-old teenager. Indeed, conducting activities of this nature are illegal; yet, there was a large public backing that having sex was a part of life that the adolescent would have missed out on. I, on the other hand, felt that it was not only ridiculous but also immoral according to my Christian beliefs.

I suppose though that my sentiments about having sex were hypocritical considering that I was having sex throughout my treatments. As a 16-year-old, I had all the natural urges that one would have; however, during the period of my life when I felt ill all day long and nothing could bring solace to me, I thought that sexual intercourse might provide some relief from the nausea. My recollections of the acts were that some of the time it helped, but most of the time, the relief was very brief. It was a never-ending sense of agony that could not be overtaken. All I wanted during these times was for someone to hold my hand, lie next to me, and show me that I was loved just like the 15 year old who desired to be touched by something other than nausea.

Chapter 19:

Closing Thoughts

Those words, those dreaded words, "You have cancer," to the layman ring in revolving thoughts of death, life's end, and unfortunate consequences. But thinking through this perspective is faulty. Today, there are revolutionary treatments, experimental approaches, and clinical trials with which one can make a conscious attempt to preserving the most important thing in this world—life. But there must be reasons why individuals choose not to go down the road of trying to extend their existence. So let's examine these viewpoints to better understand their concerns.

One common expression heard is "I'm putting it in God's hands." Each time I hear this phrase I think:

OK…but what are you going to do with your own power and God-given abilities to ensure that you are giving yourself the best chance to survive, not just for your sake, but for the sake of your friends, family, children, and others with whom you affect advantageously each and every day.

There is no question that God plays a role in everything that we do, every healing that occurs, and each miracle that takes place; yet, that is not to say that earthly acts do not also matter and influence life. God gave each human being free will along with the ability to learn and use one's brain towards making rational and logical decisions.

Having spoken to many who have come into contact with the hellish face of cancer, my perspective is different from many, maybe even most. Nevertheless, it needs to be heard so that others can know their options and no longer feel alone. It is expected that children, teenagers, and young adults have surgeries, receive chemotherapy, and/or radiation in an attempt to rid their bodies of cancerous diseases; however, a completely different approach is taken to middle-age and elderly patients. Expressions like "Well, they have lived a good life" or "It was just her time" can be heard repeated over and over and over again. Bullshit! These are the same individuals who taught us to never stop trying, don't ever give up, and do whatever it takes. So why be hypocritical when it comes to your own hardships?

Quality vs. Quantity of Life

The age-old debate revolves around the notion that once one reaches a certain age, his/her quality of life diminishes to the point that it is not worth trying to save if a serious health problem arises. I refute that argument in its entirety. Last time I checked, any life is worth saving, from one in the womb of a mother to be. "Don't give up. Don't ever give up," uttered by the great basketball coach, Jim Valvano of the North Carolina State University, never hold more weight than when it comes to battling cancer. Let me iterate that I am not trying to take away from the intolerable pain of chemotherapy, the sicknesses that result from a cancer-riddled body, or the after-effects of both. But still, life is life. There is a reason why God placed each of us here, and it is our responsibility to live up to our potential and live as long as we can to serve the needs of others in the footsteps that God laid down for us.

Proper Medical Treatment

As important as it is to develop a positive mindset to defeat cancer, it is just as critical for one to receive proper treatment. Incorrect diagnoses, undefined treatment plans, limitations from health insurance plans, and failure to research about where to receive the best possible treatment lead thousands to die every year. Each of these four areas will be addressed individually to provide a means for not becoming a victim of the *system* and instead be a winner in this ridiculous circus-like game.

343

Typically, one begins to feel sick, whether it is having flu-like or mononucleosis symptoms, trouble breathing, tiredness, pain, or organ malfunction, it is so very important that you go to the doctor immediately. Don't expect illnesses to go away by themselves or that your body will heal naturally on its own; you could be jeopardizing your life. I was fortunate enough to become diagnosed in the third stage of four, with the fourth stage of NHL being a virtual death sentence.

So you go to your doctor and nothing comes from it...go to another....go to a specialist...the best one you can find locally. If it is thought that there might be a serious health concern, begin your research efforts if you haven't already begun them. Take nothing for granted and do not rule out any possibility. Remember—Don't be a sucker in the system. I was misdiagnosed by the head oncologist at the most renowned cancer hospital in Baton Rouge, Louisiana. This goes to show you that perhaps there are specialists who know more than anyone near where you live. Needless to say, do not let geographical constraints be an issue if at all possible. Some might resist these recommendations saying, "But I have three kids in school, my husband needs me around, and I do not have the money to support those treatments." Well, find a way! What are your kids going to do without a mom or dad? What is your spouse going to do when you aren't there permanently? How much money is life worth? These troubling scenarios paint a picture that is geared towards encouraging you to have the will to get it done, and don't quit until your health is restored.

Treatment… the word by itself isn't specific, and maybe it shouldn't be for two reasons: one—there are endless possibilities for options concerning cancer treatment from surgical/laser removal of growths, radiation, chemotherapy, and a host of others; two—using the word treatment minimizes more initial shock of having cancer. If one were to say, you are going to be hooked up intravenously to a death-like toxic liquid compound, most individuals would not rush to get in line like a *Black Friday* shopping spree. So for these reasons, treatment will also be referred to within this body of work; however, I will not refrain from telling you every intimate detail of my most difficult and most rewarding experience of my life.

Treatments for cancer are carefully organized into protocols in which researchers have placed numerous drugs together so that in combination one will have a greater likelihood of eradicating cancer.

At least one would hope there is a protocol. There are two instances in which protocols are not utilized; one—the type of cancer is virtually unknown and there have not been treatments and/or experimental approaches researched; two—the oncologists with whom you are seeing are not fully qualified to treat your type of cancer and do not sufficiently have the background knowledge and previous experience working with other cancer patients who have your disease/illness.

Unfortunately, it occurs more often than one could imagine. Growing up in *Cancer Alley* in Baton Rouge, Louisiana, I have witnessed countless times that oncologists have given patients of all ages inconsistent and poorly thought-out treatment plans. The idea of doing chemotherapy on a come and go basis—meaning let's see how your body reacts/tolerates it and let's go from there. Well, whose body tolerates chemotherapy well? The exact reason for using chemotherapy is to suppress cells from replicating; in the process of killing rapidly developing cancer cells, normal growing cells die as well. Suppressing the body to remain as near death as possible is the concept behind chemotherapy, aiding to prevent cells from easily replicating. With advances in medical research, targeted treatments

346

are used to minimize the number of healthy cell loss. Thus, it is my impression that medically sound and sometimes completely experimental protocols are necessary to pursue for the sake of the patient and future patients who will develop that disease. Your efforts and tribulations shall define the extent to which you are willing to go to preserve your life, not only for you but every other being who has been, is, and will be affected for years to come.

Negative attitudes

I can do it on my own…just leave me alone. How many times are people going to ask before it becomes clearer in their heads? I am sick and tired of hearing the same old questions. Let me do this on my own. Meanwhile, thoughts enter the mind of how you have been hurt in the past by looking for assistance, relying on someone else, and giving of yourself to another just to have your hopes and needs crushed by insensitive people who were supposed to be your friends and family.

Frankly speaking though, one cannot undergo such a life-threatening and life-altering ordeal without the weight being lifted off his/her shoulders. The first step in this process is reflecting through prayer and analyzing the entire situation. We must prepare our hearts for those revelations of God's presence through our daily interactions with others. That is where God is present on earth—is each of us. If you take out a burning ember from a fire and set it nearby, you can see how the ember can only flourish in relation to other embers.

Forgetting the past that associated resentment is critical because you really do need help. Accepting that help is sometimes intolerable…that is until it works to your advantage. If you can think for one minute that others desire to help and minimize your everyday duties, you can focus where you need to—on the cancer that each day grows, manifests, and tries to overcome not only your body but your spirit. Yet, once the focus and commitment is in place, sound medical care has begun, and assistance is provided by others, it is through God's grace and one's relentless spirit that healing occurs. Never stop believing and never stop trying to defeat cancer…you are stronger than any disease.

One of my favorite authors, Thomas Merton, wrote:

We do not exist for ourselves alone, and it is only when we are fully convinced of this fact that we begin to love ourselves properly and thus also love others . . . desiring to love, accepting life as a very great gift and a great good, not because of what it gives us, but because of what it enables us to give to others. If we live for others, we will gradually discover that no one expects us to be "as gods." We will see that we are human, like everyone else, that we all have weaknesses and deficiencies, and that these limitations of ours play a most important part in all our lives. It is because of them that we need others and others need us. We are not all weak in the same spots, and so we supplement and complete one another, each one making up in himself for the lack in another.

We live and love and long for closer, deeper, and more meaningful relationships. Tragedies bring us closer to one another; however, it should not take these life changing events to change our lives. We have the power each day to choose how to live and how to love, or whether we do at all for that matter. So instead of pursuing individualistic achievements for accolades sake, let's stand up and share our joy for life while we are still living so that we can show the future of the world what a bright place it truly is.

We must embrace that we need one another. We can learn from one another.

Giving kinship, finding common ground, and discover each others' identities has ramifications far beyond our comprehension. But what is well understood are the positive effects that stem from these activities. Cancer patients are immediately cut out from communication and society in that they are different. Instead of seeing them as different, I wish that it could be understood in the sense that they are everyday people who are in a phase of their lives in which support is needed. The scale of dependency tips one way or another and thus, it is our job to provide the means to give and receive from this wonderful population.

What can we do? This question can be simply answered by saying that we must our presence as the greatest gift of all. Learn to be present when there is not much you can do physically to alleviate pain/discomfort. Be a friend of time. Moreover, gently use touch, whether at the hand, shoulder, head, or side, to replace oral communication when it is uncomfortable to communicate orally. Through touch, two become one and in turn, we can alleviate the sufferer's pain. And finally, we must become better listeners. In a world that values speeding to the next destination, patience and an

open ear are ever-valuable to console those battling cancer. Every

journey is a crossing, and having accompaniment eases the stress of

each step.

References

American Cancer Society. (2009). Detailed guide: Lymphoma, non-
Hodgkin type, *What*

  is non-Hodgkin's Lymphoma?, Retrieved July 18, 2009, from

  http://www.cancer.org/docroot/CRI/content/CRI_2_4_1X_W

  hat_Is_Non_Hodgkins_Lymphoma_32.asp?sitearea=CRI

Errett, B. (December 23, 2001). *Dying boy, 15, gets wish: losing*
virginity. Chicago Sun

  Times.

St. Jude Children's Research Hospital. (2003, Autumn). A class act.
Promise Magazine.

St. Jude Children's Research Hospital. (2007, September). *Back to*
school. Retrieved July

  13, 2009, from

  http://www.stjude.org/stjude/v/index.jsp?vgnextoid=b20ab91

  d7ccd4110VgnVCM1000001e0215acRCRD&vgnextchannel

  =a525aab5033c1110VgnVCM1000001e0215acRCRD&

Smith, M. (2009, February 12). *Web cam helps cancer patient not*
miss a beat. Retrieved

July 18, 2009, from

http://www.wtop.com/?nid=25&sid=1600094

Appendix A

Wong-Baker FACES
Pain Rating Scale

English

 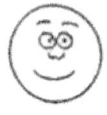 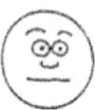  

0	2	4	6	8	10
No Hurt	Hurts Little Bit	Hurts Little More	Hurts Even More	Hurts Whole Lot	Hurts Worst

Escala de CARAS de Wong-Baker
para manifestar la intensidad del dolor

Spanish

 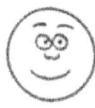    

0	2	4	6	8	10
No Duele	Duele Poquito	Duele un poco más	Duele aún más	Duele Mucho	Duele Mucho más

Appendix B:

Wish-Granting Organizations

- **Adventures For Wish Kids - Ohio**

  http://www.afwkids.org/

  Provides continuing support and lasting memories for children and adolescents with life threatening illness and their families.

- **Angelwish**

  http://www.angelwish.org/

  We are going to remove all the obstacles that have stood in your way of helping others, especially children and their families that are living with HIV/AIDS.

- **Believe In Tomorrow National Children's Foundation**

  http://www.believeintomorrow.org/

  Our programs and services help children with life-threatening illnesses believe in hope, joy and the promise of tomorrow. Our foundation is dedicated to improving the quality of life for critically ill children and their families through three unique programs. Serving over 38,000 children each year, we have become a national leader in pediatric support services that help to ease pain, reduce loneliness and bring joy to children throughout their treatment process.

- **Canadian Centre for Abuse Awareness**

  http://www.ccfaa.com

Grants non-travel wishes and programs to severely abused and neglected children.

- **Central Illinois Dream Factory**
  http://www.dreamfactoryci.com/
  Grants dreams to children in the Central Illinois area (75 mile radius of Peoria, Illinois), who are between the ages of 3 and 18 years who have been diagnosed with critical or chronic illnesses.

- **Chef David's Kids**
  http://www.chefdavidskids.com/
  We help children afflicted with any form of terminal illness such as cancer, leukemia, and pediatric HIV. We also help with neglected and abused children. We have handled thousands of interactions and wishes for children in the last ten years and have never failed to help when needed, no matter how many times a child needs us.

- **Children's Wish Foundation International**
  http://www.childrenswish.org/
  Children's Wish will fulfill the favorite wish for any child not expected to reach age 18. Each wish, truly the child's own, must be completed while the child is healthy enough to fully enjoy it. The immediate family is included in the wish fulfillment, so that the child and family will share in the experience and create happy memories together.

- **Children's Wish Foundation of Canada—Canada**

  http://www.childrenswish.ca/

  This organization with 12 provincial Chapter Offices from coast to coast is dedicated to fulfilling a favorite wish for children afflicted with a high risk, life-threatening illness.

- **Dial-a-Dream—United Kingdom**

  http://www.dial-a-dream.co.uk/

  This organization strives to make Dreams a reality for children suffering a life threatening or debilitating illness, and thereby enabling them to continue their fight against their illness.

- **Dream-A-Wish Foundation—Florida**

  http://www.dream-a-wish.org/

  Dream-A-Wish has a goal to stop the clock and give Central Florida families a few quality hours away from pain, worry, and stress. This happens when we complete a dream and give them a week of wonderful memories to last a lifetime.

- **Dream Come True—Pennsylvania**

  http://www.dreamcometrue.org/

  Dream Come True seeks to fulfill the dreams of children who are seriously, chronically, and terminally ill and reside in the greater Lehigh Valley area of Pennsylvania.

- **Dreams Come True**

  http://www.dreamscometrue.org/

  Provides wishes for children battling life-threatening illnesses in Northeast Florida and Southeast Georgia. All children between the ages of two and a half and eighteen who have been diagnosed with a life-threatening illness and either live or are treated in Northeast Florida or Southeast Georgia, including Shands Gainesville, are eligible for a dreams. Children must be referred by their physician and have all activities approved.

- **Dream Factory**
  http://www.dreamfactoryinc.com/
  The Dream Factory grants dreams to children diagnosed with critical or chronic illnesses who are 3 through 18 years of age.

- **Dream Factory of Greater Kansas City**
  http://www.kcdream.org/
  Grants wishes to seriously or chronically ill children aged 3 to 18 who live in the greater Kansas City area.

- **Dream Foundation**
  http://www.dreamfoundation.com/
  Dream Foundation is a national wish-granting organization who grants the wishes of terminally ill adults aged 18 to 65.

- **Dream Lives On - Alaska**
  http://thedreamliveson.org/
  Adults, age 18 years and older, who have been diagnosed with a year or less to live.

- **Fairygodmother Foundation**

  http://www.fairygodmother.org/

  Fairygodmother Foundation make wishes come true for individuals (18 and older) and loved ones in their time of greatest need by turning dreams into reality.

- **Give Kids the World**

  http://www.gktw.org/

  This organization is not a wish-granting organization in the strictest sense. Rather, it works with other wish foundations to send children with life threatening illnesses to the Central Florida area. Every child that comes to Give Kids The World does so with the sponsorship of another wish granting organization. It has served children from all 50 states and more than 45 countries.

- **Happiness Unlimited - New Jersey**

  http://www.happiness-unlimited.org/

  A unique, one-of-a-kind, wish-fulfillment program for adults with cancer.

- **Her Heart's Wish**

  http://www.herheartswish.org/

  National organization dedicated to granting the wishes of adult women who are facing terminal illness.

- **High Hopes Foundation of New Hampshire, Inc.**

  http://www.highhopesnh.org/

Dedicated to granting the wishes of New Hampshire's severely and chronically ill children between the ages of 3 and 18.

- **Hopes & Dreams Foundation of Oklahoma**
  http://www.normand.org/gigi/
  A non-profit, volunteer organization which was founded to inspire children who have terminal illnesses, life-threatening medical conditions, or are physically challenged. The main goal of HOPES and DREAMS is to enrich the lives of the children in our foundation by sending them, as often as possible to events in the State of Oklahoma. These events are choosen for our children by our children! HOPES and DREAMS works hard to get tickets, passes, autographed pictures, and personal contacts for our children.

- **Hopes & Dreams - United Kingdom**
  http://www.hopesdreams.org/
  Has a goal to fulfill the dreams of terminally and chronically ill children and young adults whether it be meeting their favorite singer or band, going to see their chosen football team, and meeting the players, going to see a show, visiting a theme park etc.

- **HopeKids**
  http://www.hopekids.org/
  Provides ongoing events & activities and a powerful, unique support community for children with cancer and other life-threatening medical conditions.

- **Indiana Children's Wish Foundation**

  http://www.indianachildrenswishfund.org/

  The Indiana Children's Wish Fund grants the wishes of special Indiana Children who suffer from a life-threatening illness. These children are between the ages of 3-18.

- **Jason's Dreams For Kids**

  http://www.jasonsdreamsforkids.com/

  The organization is devoted to granting wishes to children diagnosed with life-threatening illnesses. Bringing a little happiness and putting a few smiles on these children's faces is our goal - and hopefully, their parents faces, too!

- **Kidd's Kids—Texas**

  http://www.kiddskids.com/

  This is a non profit organization within KHKS-FM Radio which each year takes children with special medical needs on the trip of a lifetime to Walt Disney World! Children selected for the Kidd's Kids trip are between the ages of 5 and 11, suffer from a chronic, terminal, or traumatic illness, reside in the Dallas/Fort Worth area, and demonstrate a financial need.

- **Kids Wish Network**

  http://www.kidswishnetwork.com/

  Kids Wish Network is a nonprofit charitable organization whose sole mission is to grant wishes to children with life-threatening illnesses. We're always looking for ways to provide unique services for sick children and their families that they

361

are not likely to find anywhere else. Kids Wish Network has developed a funeral assistance program to assist the families of "our kids" who have passed away.

- **The Joshua Foundation—United Kingdom**
  http://www.thejoshuafoundation.co.uk/
  Provides holidays and experiences for children and their families where the child is diagnosed with terminal cancer.

- **Make-a-Wish Foundation of America**
  http://www.wish.org/
  This organization which serves all 50 states, Guam, and Puerto Rico grants wishes to children in the United States with terminal illnesses or life-threatening medical conditions that create the probability the children will not survive beyond their 18th year.

- **Make-a-Wish Foundation of Canada—Canada**
  http://www.makeawish.ca/
  This chapter which serves various regions in Canada seeks to fulfill the special wishes of children under the age of 18 who have life-threatening illnesses.

- **Make-a-Wish Foundation of India—India**
  http://makeawish.indo.net/
  This chapter which serves those in India helps children suffering from life threatening diseases realize their heart's desire.

- **Make-A-Wish Foundation of Wisconsin**

  http://www.wisconsin.wish.org/

- **The Marty Lyons Foundation**

  http://www.martylyonsfoundation.org/

  Established to fulfill the special wishes of children aged three to seventeen years old, who have been diagnosed as having a terminal or life threatening illness by providing and arranging special wish requests. The principal office is in New York, but the Foundation also operates chapters in New Jersey, New York, Massachusetts, Connecticut, Maryland, Pennsylvania, South Carolina, Georgia and Florida.

- **Never Too Late**

  http://www.nevertoolate.org/

  Staffed by a passionate group of volunteers who donate their time and talents to help make the dreams and wishes of the forgotten elderly and terminally ill adults come true.

- **Round Table Children's Wish - United Kingdom**

  http://www.rtcw.org/

  Grant Wishes to children suffering from life-threatening illnesses.

- **Silver Lining Foundation**

  http://www.silverliningfoundation.org/

  Among other things, the Silver Lining Foundation provides

wishes for children with cancer while their are receiving treatment.

- **A Special Wish Foundation, Inc.**
  http://www.spwish.org/
  This organization's mission is to enhance the quality of life for those children/adolescents (under 20 years of age) who have a life-threatening or terminal disorder by allowing their special wish to become reality. It has 21 chapters throughout the U.S. as well as a chapter in Moscow, Russia.

- **Starlight Children's Foundation**
  http://www.starlight.org/
  This organization is dedicated to brightening the lives of seriously ill children through wish granting and state-of-the-art in-hospital entertainment. It has a network of chapters located in the United States, the United Kingdom, Australia, and Canada.

- **Starlight Children's Foundation Canada - Canada**
  http://www.starlightcanada.org/
  This chapter which serves Canada is dedicated to brightening the lives of seriously ill children through wish granting and state-of-the-art in-hospital entertainment.

- **Sunshine Foundation**
  http://www.sunshinefoundation.org/
  This organization which serves those across the United States

fulfills dreams and wishes of chronically ill, terminally ill handicapped and abused children. The majority of wishes the Sunshine Foundation fulfills are to visit a Central Florida attraction.

- **Sunshine Foundation of Canada—Canada**
  http://sunshine.wwdc.com/
  This foundation allows children with a severe physical disability or life-threatening illness to have a chance to see their once-in-a-lifetime dream come true.

- **Tender Wishes—Canada**
  http://www.tenderwishes.org/
  This organization grants wishes to children between the ages of 2 and 18, who have a life-threatening illness, and reside in the Regional Municipality of Niagara.

- **United Special Sportsmen Alliance**
  http://www.childswish.com/
  A non-profit Christian organization that routinely coordinates with other caring organizations worldwide in fulfilling a dream wish. If you know of a child [or adult] who is terminally ill or disabled and would like to go on a FREE DREAM HUNT, FISHING TRIP AND CAMPING OR CANOEING please contact U.S.S.A and we will try to fulfill their "Dream Wish." Working with deer, elk, turkey, bear, pheasant farms, and property owners as well as, preserves and ranches has made our hunting, fishing trips and outdoor adventures known nationwide.

- **When You Wish Upon A Star—United Kingdom**

  http://www.whenyouwishuponastar.org.uk/

  Aims to fulfill the wishes of children with life threatening and terminal illnesses.

- **Willow Foundation—United Kingdom**

  http://www.willowfoundation.org.uk/

  A charity dedicated to improving the quality of life of seriously ill adults aged 16 to 40 by organising and funding a 'special day' of their choice. Special days give young people with life-threatening or life-limiting conditions a chance to escape the difficulties of their daily routine and share quality time with family and friends while pursuing an activity they can all enjoy.

- **Wishing Star—Idaho and Eastern Washington State**

  http://www.wishingstar.org/

  This organization grants wishes to children age 3-19 with life threatening diseases in Idaho and Eastern Washington State.

- **Wish Upon a Star—California**

  http://www.wishuponastar.org/

  Our assistance is available to children in the state of California. Most often children are referred to our program by medical staff working in the major Children's and University Hospitals. A statewide network of law enforcement personnel and community volunteers allows Wish Upon A Star to operate quickly, regardless of a child's location or circumstance.

- **A Wish With Wings—Texas**

  http://www.awishwithwings.org/

  This organization grants wishes to children with life-threatening or catastrophic illness between the ages of 3 and 17, who reside or receive treatment in the State of Texas or out of State with Board Members' approval.

- **Wishing Well Foundation**

  http://www.wishingwellusa.org/

  The Wishing Well Foundation will consider the wish of any child with a life threatening illness from ages 3 to 18. The Wishing Well Foundation receives referrals from doctors, nurses, and people just like you! Many of the wishes are for trips to theme parks or a special day with a special someone . . . perhaps a celebrity or hero. The wish can be most complex or very simple.

Index

6-MP- 6-Mercaptopurine

Ara-C – Cytarabine, also known as cytosine arabinoside

Bone Marrow Aspirate (BMA)

Bone Marrow Biopsy (BMB)

Complete Blood Count (CBC)

Central line (Hickman, sub-quetaneous portacathe)

Central Nervous System (CNS)

Chemoreceptor trigger zone (CTZ)

chemotherapy induced nausea and vomiting (CINV)

CT Scan- computed tomography scan

CTX

Cyclophosphamide (Cytoxan)

daunorubicine

dexomethosone (Dex)

Federal Drug Administration (FDA)

intramuscular (IM)

Intratheical (IT)

Intravenous (IV)

Leucovorin – Folinic Acid; typically administered as an ajuvant used in cancer

      chemotherapy treatment

lumbar puncture (LP)

Methotrexate (MTX)

Magnetic Resonance Imaging (MRI)

Non-Hodgkin's Lymphoma (NHL)

orally-disintegrating tablets (ODT)

PO- By mouth

Prednisone - a corticosteroid that is used for various purposes including as an

      immunosuppressant

Radiation therapy- also known as radio therapy; it is used as pallatative therapy for local

      disease control

SQ (sub-quetaneous)

Vincristin – leurocristine; side effects include neuropathy--loss of reflexes

VP-16 – etoposide phosphate;

X-Ray – Rontagen Ray

Resources

Medical

www.survivorshipguidelines.org

Educational

www.reedmartin.com

www.nichcy.org

www.memorybridge.org

Academic

www.ortliebfoundation.com